Glossary of Oral and Maxillofacial Implants

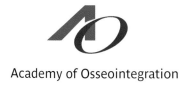

Academy of Osseointegration

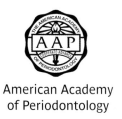

American Academy
of Periodontology

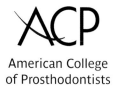

American College
of Prosthodontists

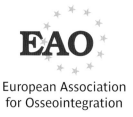

European Association
for Osseointegration

Editor-in-Chief

W. R. Laney

Glossary of Oral and Maxillofacial Implants

Section Editors:

N. Broggini
D. Buser
D. L. Cochran
L. T. Garcia
W. V. Giannobile
E. Hjørting-Hansen
T. D. Taylor

Co-Editors:

J. A. Cirelli
K. Dula
R. E. Jung
R. T. Yanase

Quintessence Publishing Co, Ltd
Berlin, Chicago, Tokyo, Barcelona, Beijing, Istanbul, London,
Milan, Moscow, New Delhi, Paris, Prague, São Paulo, Seoul, and Warsaw

German National Library CIP Data
The German National Library has listed this publication in the German National Bibliography. Detailed bibliographical data are available on the Internet at http://dnb.ddb.de.

 © 2007 Quintessence Publishing Co, Ltd
Ifenpfad 2-4, 12107 Berlin,
www.quintessenz.de

Initiator: A. Ammann (QPC Berlin)
Coordination: Ä. Klebba (QPC Berlin)
Editing: L. Bywaters (QPC Chicago)
Illustrations: U. Drewes (www.drewes.ch)
Production: J. Richter (QPC Berlin)
Printing: Bosch-Druck GmbH
                  (www.bosch-druck.de)

Printed in Germany
ISBN: 978-3-938947-00-5

Acknowledgement

The authors thank Ms. Ute Drewes for her beautiful artwork and illustrations. We also thank Ms. E.F. Davis for her excellent support and outstanding commitment during the entire editing process.

Sources of figures

The majority of the figures in this book were computer-generated by Ms. U. Drewes. These illustrations are not labeled with a source. The remaining figures were reproduced from previous publications with permission from the respective authors or publishers. These figures are labeled with a source.

Foreword

The preparation of the Glossary of Oral and Maxillofacial Implants represents a crucial step towards harmonizing the terminology employed worldwide by clinicians, researchers and academics who work in this field and establishing a solid basis for mutual understanding.

The International Team for Implantology (ITI) has no hesitation in endorsing this valuable work and congratulates its author, Prof. Dr. William R. Laney, his co-contributors and advisors on producing such an extensive, accurate and considered work.

The aim of the ITI is to promote and disseminate knowledge on all aspects of implant dentistry and related tissue regeneration. As it demonstrated with the ITI Treatment Guide series, the ITI is keen to support the development of practical tools for professionals in this field. As a work that lays the foundations for a shared vocabulary, the Glossary of Oral and Maxillofacial Implants is sure to become an indispensable tool for every professional fascinated by the vast array of terminology in the field and who also has the desire to employ it accurately and meaningfully.

This volume does not aspire to the impossible task to cover all terms in this field. It has, however, selected around 2000 of the most commonly used terms from various areas of implant dentistry.

The ITI is proud to have been involved in the development of this volume and is happy to recommend it as a standard work from which every professional in the field can benefit.

Congratulations on a job well done.

Dieter Weingart   *Daniel Buser*
ITI President   Chairman,
ITI Education Committee

V

Preface

As the field of implant dentistry has grown internationally, so has the need for a common implant language. With new developments and technology has come an increasingly diverse and complex literature. For clinicians, educators, and researchers alike, it is time to bring universal consistency to the terminology of implant dentistry.

One component of the multimedia, multi-language series by the Quintessence Publishing Company, entitled Dynamics in Implant Dentistry, includes an illustrated glossary that provides a broadly based multidisciplinary introduction to scientific terminology pertinent to the field. From a thorough review of implant textbooks and peer-reviewed periodical literature, some 5000 terms were distilled for consideration. Approximately 2000 of these were selected for inclusion and defined by co-authors representing an interdisciplinary variety of implant-related interests, including surgery, radiology, hard and soft tissue biology, periodontics, prosthodontics, implant componentry, research methodology and statistics, biomechanics and ceramics.

Closely related to the expansion of implant clinical practice has been the competitive technical development and marketing activities by manufacturers of implant system components, instruments, and devices. While acknowledging that these products are essential to the expansion of implant dentistry, it is important to note that the intended aim of this glossary is to focus on collaborative science and art as the basis for implant therapy advancement and to minimize emphasis on commercial hardware technology and terminology.

The dedicated members of the Editorial Board who have compiled and written this first-edition represent the expertise of essential disciplines comprising the broad spectrum of implant dentistry. To the following contributors, I extend my heartfelt thanks and appreciation for their participation, cooperation, and especially their well-recognized expertise: Prof. Dr. Daniel Buser, Dr. Nina Broggini, Dr. Karl Dula, Prof. Dr. Erik Hjørting-Hansen, Prof. Dr. William Giannobile, Dr. Joni Cirelli, Prof. Dr. Lily Garcia, Dr. Roy Yanase, Prof. Dr. David Cochran, Dr. Ronald Jung and Prof. Dr. Thomas Taylor. In addition, Drs. Peter C. O'Brien and Thomas G. Wilson, Jr. have contributed considerably to the glossary in support of the co-authors.

Without the profound interest and support of the International Team for Implantology, this glossary could not have progressed.

A work of this complexity and magnitude must involve the collaboration of capable support personnel. Ms. Ute Drewes has contributed her artistic skills to the creation of illuminative illustrations. The daily tasks of compiling and editing database input have been timely and extraordinarily accomplished by Ms. Elizabeth Floyd Davis (USA) and Ms. Änne Klebba, Quintessence Publishing, Berlin. Ms. Sandra Fielitz provided secretarial support in Quintessence Berlin and efficiently managed the laborious task of preparing the initial database from which the included terms were selected. The final review, coordination and editing of terms was superbly accomplished by Ms. Lisa Bywaters, Senior Editor, and her staff at Quintessence Publishing, Chicago. This publication was conceived and very capably managed by Mr. Alexander Ammann, Project Di-

rector of Quintessence Berlin. Mr. Bernd Burkart, head of the Quintessence Berlin production department, coordinated and directed all production activities. The dedication, perseverance, and cooperation of the entire Quintessence Publishing Company staff have been exemplary.

It is anticipated that the *Glossary of Oral and Maxillofacial Implants* will become a practical education and communications tool for those students and practitioners who have or will have an interest in implant dentistry. Nonetheless, this print resource should be considered a work in progress. New knowledge will continue to emerge and with it the need for additional terms, revision of those existing, and deletion of those that are redundant or obsolete.

William R. Laney, DMD, MS

William R. Laney

Editor and Authors

Oral and Maxillofacial Surgery/Diagnostics/Anatomy/X-Ray

Authors
Daniel Buser, DMD, Prof., Dr. med. dent.
Professor/Chair, Department of Oral Surgery
and Stomatology
School of Dental Medicine
University of Bern
Freiburgstrasse 7
3010 Bern, SWITZERLAND
daniel.buser@zmk.unibe.ch

Nina Broggini, DMD, MS, Dr. med. dent.
Department of Oral Surgery and Stomatology
School of Dental Medicine
University of Bern
Freiburgstrasse 7
3010 Bern, SWITZERLAND
nina.broggini@zmk.unibe.ch

Private Practice:
Studio Borsa Broggini Lanfranchini
Via Stazione 1
6828 Balerna, SWITZERLAND
studiobbl@ticino.com

Co-Author
Karl Dula, PD, Dr. med. dent.
Chair, Section of Dental Radiology
Department of Oral Surgery and Stomatology
School of Dental Medicine
University of Bern
Freiburgstrasse 7
3010 Bern, SWITZERLAND
karl.dula@zmk.unibe.ch

Biomedicine/Biomaterials

Author
Erik Hjørting-Hansen, Prof., Dr. odont.
Department of Oral and Maxillofacial Surgery
School of Dentistry and University Hospital
(Rigshospitalet)
University of Copenhagen
Norre Alle 20
2200 Copenhagen N, DENMARK
erik.boneart@mail.dk

Periodontics

Author
William V. Giannobile DDS, D. Med. Sc.
Najjar Professor of Dentistry
Director
Michigan Center for Oral Health Research
University of Michigan
24 Frank Lloyd Wright Drive
Lobby M, Box 422
Ann Arbor, MI 48106, USA
wgiannob@umich.edu

Co-Author
Joni Augusto Cirelli, DDS, PhD
Research Fellow, Department of Periodontics
and Oral Medicine
School of Dentistry
University of Michigan
1011 N. University Avenue
Ann Arbor, MI 48109, USA
cirelli@umich.edu

Prosthodontics

Author/Editor-in-Chief
William R. Laney, DMD, MS
Professor Emeritus
Division of Prosthodontics
Department of Dental Specialties
Mayo Clinic College of Medicine
Rochester, MN 55905, USA
quinjomi@aol.com

Contributors
Peter C. O'Brien, PhD
Professor of Biostatistics
Division of Biostatistics
Department of Health Sciences Research
Mayo Clinic College of Medicine
Rochester, MN 55905, USA
obrien@mayo.edu

Thomas G. Wilson, Jr., DDS
Private Practice of Periodontics
5465 Blair Road, Suite 200
Dallas, TX 75231, USA
tom@tgwperio.com

Implant Componentry

Author
Lily T. Garcia, DDS, MS
Professor/Chair, Department of Prosthodontics
University of Texas Health Science Center at
San Antonio
7703 Floyd Curl Drive, MSC 7912
San Antonio, TX 78229-3900, USA
garcialt@uthscsa.edu

Co-Author
Roy T. Yanase, DDS
Clinical Professor, Continuing Education and
Advanced Education in Prosthodontics
University of Southern California
School of Dentistry
22330 Hawthorne Boulevard, Suite 316
Torrance, CA 90505-2590, USA
rtydds@aol.com

Biometry/Statistics/Research/Methodology

Author
David L. Cochran, DDS, MS, PhD, MMSci
Professor, Department of Periodontics
MSC 7894
University of Texas Health Science
Center at San Antonio
7703 Floyd Curl Drive
San Antonio, TX 78229-3900, USA
cochran@uthscsa.edu

Co-Author
Ronald E. Jung, Dr. med. dent.
Assistant Professor, Clinic for Fixed
and Removable Prosthodontics
Center for Dental and Oral Medicine
and Cranio-Maxillofacial Surgery
University of Zurich
Plattenstrasse 11
8032 Zurich, SWITZERLAND
jung@zzmk.unizh.ch

Biomechanics/Ceramics

Author
Thomas D. Taylor, DDS, MSD
Professor/Chair,
Department of Reconstructive Sciences
University of Connecticut School
of Dental Medicine
263 Farmington Avenue
Farmington, CT 06030-1615, USA
ttaylor@nso.uchc.edu

A
B
C
D
E
F
G
H
I
J
K
L
M
N
O
P
Q
R
S
T
U
V
W
X Y
Z

A

Abscess Pathologic process that is an enclosed collection of purulent exudates (pus) in tissues, organs, or confined spaces in the body. Signs of infection, swelling, and inflammation are typical.   See also: *Acute abscess; Chronic abscess; Gingival abscess; Periodontal abscess; Residual abscess.*

Absorbable See: *Bioabsorbable material.*

Absorption Uptake of substances into or across tissues (eg, skin, mucosa, intestine, or renal tubules).

Abutment Tooth, tooth root, or implant component that serves as support and/or retention for a dental prosthesis.[1] See also: *Anatomic healing abutment; Angled/angulated abutment; CAD/CAM abutment; Castable abutment; Ceramic abutment; Healing abutment; Nonangled abutment; Nonrotating abutment; Prefabricated abutment; Preparable abutment; Standard abutment; Temporary abutment; Transmucosal abutment; UCLA abutment.*

Screw design of a. Prosthetic implant component manufactured with threads at the apical portion of the element. This term refers to the manufacture of a specific thread pattern unique to a particular implant company.

Tightness of a. Amount of clamping force present within the body of an abutment screw following placement. See also: *Preload.*

Abutment clamp Instrument used to handle or hold the implant abutment. The concave design is such that when engaged, the clamp fits circumferentially around the component.

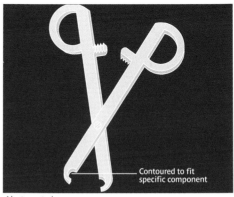

Contoured to fit specific component

Abutment clamp.

Abutment connection Act of connecting an abutment to an endosseous implant.[2,3] See also: *External abutment connection; Internal abutment connection; Morse taper connection.*

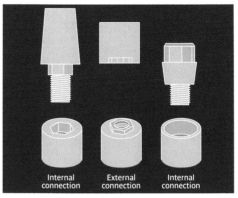

Internal connection External connection Internal connection

Abutment connection.
(Redrawn from Yanase and Preston[3] with perission.)

Abutment-implant interface Common contact surface area between an implant abutment and the supporting implant.[3]

Abutment screw Single-piece implant component with a threaded apical portion that can be connected directly to the implant. No additional screw is required to connect and secure the abutment component.

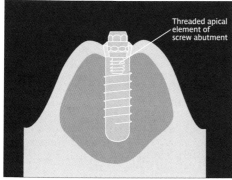

Threaded apical element of screw abutment

Abutment screw.

Access hole Opening in a replacement tooth's occlusal or lingual surface of an implant-retained prosthesis that provides entrance for abutment or prosthesis screw placement or removal.[3]

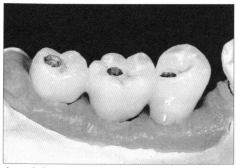

Access hole.
(Reprinted from Watzek[4] with permission.)

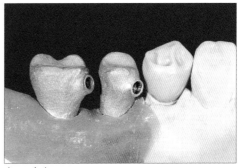

Access hole.
(Reprinted from Watzek[4] with permission.)

Acellular Limited in or devoid of cells.

Acellular dermal allograft Skin graft made of a thin split-thickness of dermis that has undergone a tissue-preparation process to remove cellular material.

Acid-etched implant External surface of an implant body that has been modified by the chemical action of an acidic medium. The subtractive surface is intended to enhance osseointegration.

Acid etching Act of modifying an implant surface by exposure to an acidic medium with the intention of enhancing osseointegration. See also: *Etching*.

Acquired immunity Specialized form of immunity involving antibodies and lymphocytes. Active immunity develops after exposure to a suitable agent (eg, by an attack of a disease or by injection of antigens), and passive immunity occurs with transfer of antibodies or lymphocytes from an immune donor.

Acquired immunodeficiency syndrome See: *AIDS*.

Acrylic crown   See: *Acrylic restoration*.

Acrylic resin   Thermoplastic resin produced by polymerizing esters of acrylic or methyl-methacrylate acids.

Acrylic restoration   Tooth or other prosthetic restoration fabricated from acrylic resin, such as an acrylic crown.

Actinobacillus actinomycetemcomitans   Gram-negative, fermentative, nonmotile, coccoid or rod-shaped bacterium of the family *Pasteurellaceae*, part of the normal mammalian microflora. This bacterium has been associated with periodontal infections and, in particular, early-onset, aggressive forms of periodontal disease.

Acute abscess   Abscess of relatively short duration, typically producing local swelling, inflammation, and pain.

Acute infection   Infection with a rapid onset and usually a severe course.[5]   See also: *Infection*.

Additive surface treatment   Implant surface modification created by the addition of material. Surface modification may also be accomplished by subtractive surface treatment.   Compare: *Substracted implant surface*.

Adhesive   Intervening substance used to unite adjoining surfaces. In maxillofacial prosthetics, adhesives have been used for border adaptation, marginal seal, and the retention of facial, auricular, nasal, or orbital prostheses. Systems commonly used include biphase adhesive tape and medical-grade adhesives.[6,7]

Adhesive retention   See: *Cementation*.

Adjunctive treatment   Supplementary therapeutic procedure to augment a main therapeutic procedure in an additive, usually incremental, manner.

Adjustable attachment system   Stud-shaped attachment in which the stud (easily replaced) serves as the patrix, and the matrix consists of a metal housing. The base of the patrix can be cast-to or soldered as part of a coping, and the matrix can be incorporated into the dental prosthesis. The patrix is adjustable using a special tool to modify the spread of the patrix width.[8,9]

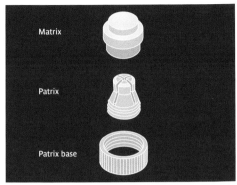

Adjustable attachment system.
(Redrawn from Staubli and Bagley[9] with permission.)

Adjustment   Modification of a tooth or prosthetic restoration to improve its appearance, fit, or function.[10]

AIDS   Acronym for *acquired immunodeficiency syndrome*, caused by HIV (human immunodeficiency virus), that leaves the body vulnerable to a host of life-threatening illnesses. There is no cure for AIDS, but treatment with antiviral medication can suppress symptoms. The virus attacks selected cells of the immune, nervous, and other systems, impairing their proper function and rendering the subject highly vulnerable to life-threatening conditions (eg, *Pneumocystis carinii pneumonia*) and those that can become life threatening (eg, *Kaposi sarcoma*). Oral lesions may include necrotizing ulcerative gingivitis (NUG), necrotized ulcerative periodontitis (NUP), linear gingival erythema (LGE), candidiasis, hairy leukoplakia, herpes simplex, and rapidly progressive periodontitis.

A

Alendronate sodium   Oral bisphosphonate used in the treatment of different types of osteoporosis with a reasonably high degree of treatment success in prevention of fractures of the vertebral column.

Algae   See: *Calcified algae.*

Algipore   See: *Calcified algae; Porous marine-derived coralline hydroxyapatite.*

Alkaline phosphatase   Enzyme found in high concentrations in osteoblasts; commonly located on cytoplasmic processes extending into the osteoid. The level of alkaline phosphatase in serum is a systemic indicator for bone formation.

Allodynia   Pain resulting from a nonnoxious stimulus that does not normally provoke pain.

Allogeneic bone graft   Graft between genetically dissimilar members of the same species. Iliac cancellous bone and marrow, freeze-dried bone allograft (FDBA), and demineralized freeze-dried bone allograft (DFDBA) are available commercially from tissue banks. Called also *allograft.*

Allograft   Graft between genetically dissimilar members of the same species.[11,12]   See also: *Acellular dermal allograft; Allogeneic bone graft; Soft tissue augmentation.*

Integration with a.   Independent of allograft or bone substitute use for osseous reconstruction, implants will always have newly formed host bone in juxtaposition to the implants as part of the process of osseointegration.

Alloplast   Inorganic, synthetic, or inert foreign material implanted into tissue.[11,12]

Alloplastic graft   Graft material such as hydroxyapatite (HA), tricalcium phosphate (TCP), polymethylmethacrylate (PMMA) and hydroxyethyl-methacrylate (HEMA) polymer, or bioactive glass that is derived either synthetically or from a foreign, inert source.   See also: *Alloplast.*

Aluminum oxide   Oxide ceramic (Al_2O_3) used in single-crystal form as implant material. Because it is biocompatible and has a hardness similar to that of the gem sapphire, it has been called *single-crystal sapphire*. Aluminum oxide has been replaced by titanium as the material of choice for implants.

Alveolar   Related to the alveolar process, the maxillary or mandibular ridge of bone that supports the roots of teeth.

Alveolar atrophy   Decrease in the volume of the alveolar process occurring after tooth loss, decreased function, and/or localized overloading from an improperly fitting removable partial or complete denture.[13]

Alveolar bone   That part of the maxilla or mandible comprising the tooth-bearing and/or supporting part of the jawbones. It consists of cortical plates, the vestibular plate being the thinnest, and trabecular bone. See also: *Atrophic alveolar bone; Cancellous bone.*

Quality of a. b.   Of major importance to the outcome of implant placement, bone quality has been categorized in a number of classification systems, illustrating the variance in relative volume of compact cortical bone and trabecular bone. Although it is often used, the term *bone quality* is a misnomer; a more correct term would be *bone density*. A popular and often-quoted classification was originally proposed by Lekholm and Zarb (1985). *Type 1* refers to homogenous compact bone of high density but low vascularity; hence not an ideal clinical situation. *Types 2* and *3* describe bone that still has a dense cortical plate but also has a cancellous portion with good vascularity for ideal implant placement and stability. *Type 4* describes inadequate density, and caution in its use for implant placement is warranted.[14]

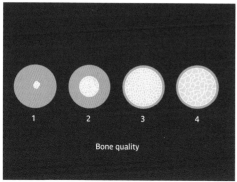

Quality of alveolar bone.
(Redrawn from Lekholm and Zarb[14] with permission.)

Quantity of a. b. Of major importance to the outcome of implant placement, bone volume at a given implant site ideally should be at least 10 mm in vertical dimension and 6 mm in horizontal dimension.[15]

Alveolar distraction osteogenesis Augmentation procedure involving the surgical mobilization, transport, and fixation of an alveolar bone segment. A mechanical distraction device allows a gradual, controlled displacement of the mobile bone segment at an ideal rate of 0.4 mm a day. Following the desired augmentation, the device is left in place for 3 to 4 weeks for consolidation of the newly formed bone.[16] See also: *Distraction osteogenesis (DO)*.

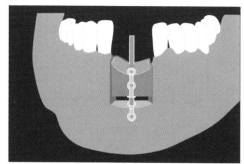

Alveolar distraction osteogenesis.
(Redrawn from Chin[16] with permission.)

Alveolar mucosa Mucosa covering the basal part of the alveolar process and continuing into the vestibulum and floor of the mouth without demarcation. In contrast to attached gingiva, alveolar mucosa is nonkeratinized, mobile, and has a thin lamina propria, numerous elastic fibers, and a distinct submucosa. It is a dark red tissue, movable, and loosely attached to the periosteum. The alveolar mucosa is coronally separated from the gingiva by a line called the *mucogingival junction*.

Alveolar nerve Either of the superior alveolar nerve branches of the maxillary nerve of the second division of the trigeminal nerve (*rami alveolares superiores posteriores, ramus alveolaris superior medius, and ramus alveolaris superior anteriores*). Supplies sensory innervation to the maxillary molars, the premolars, or the canine and incisors, respectively. The inferior alveolar nerve (*nervus alveolaris inferior*) is the largest branch of the mandibular nerve of the third division of the trigeminal nerve or cranial nerve V, which supplies sensory innervation to the mandibular teeth, lower lip, and chin. Descending between the sphenomandibular ligament and mandibular ramus, the inferior alveolar nerve enters the medial aspect of the mandible by way of the mandibular foramen and continues anteriorly through the mandibular canal, first forming the inferior dental plexus that supplies sensory innervation to the molars and premolars. Continuing anteriorly to the mental foramen, it then divides into two terminal branches: the mental nerve *(nervus mentalis)* which branches off at the level of the premolars and exits the mental foramen, supplying the sensory branches of the lower lip and chin; and the incisive branch, which supplies the canines and incisors. Other branches of the mandibular nerve include the mylohyoid nerve *(nervus mylohyoideus)*, which supplies the mylohyoideus muscle and the anterior belly of the digastricus.[17]

Alveolar process Ridge of maxillary or mandibular bone supporting the roots of erupted teeth and unerupted, developing tooth buds.

Alveolar reconstruction Surgical reconstruction of an atrophic alveolar ridge that does not allow for simultaneous implant placement because of the extent of bone deficiency. Ridge defects are present following long-standing edentulism, trauma, tumor resection, or infection. Localized defects are treated with autogenous block grafts from intraoral donor sites and often combined with particulate autogenous bone, bone substitutes, and/or barrier membranes. More extensive defects require extraoral autogenous block grafts, which offer the greatest amount of augmentation volume and stability. In vertical reconstruction, distraction osteogenesis could be an alternative to onlay grafting.

Alveolar ridge Osseous part of the mandible and maxilla remaining after removal of teeth; ie, alveolar process. This entity usually becomes atrophic when not loaded or when loaded in an unphysiologic way (eg, removable partial or complete dentures). The transfer of forces through implants can maintain ridge volume and thereby avoid atrophy.

    Classification of a. r. Several alveolar bone morphologic classification systems exist. The most classic and frequently-used system – proposed by Cawood and Howell – describes potential denture-bearing bone as *Class I*: dentate; *Class II*: immediately postextraction; *Class III*: well-rounded ridge form that has adequate height and width; *Class IV*: knife-edge ridge form, adequate in height but inadequate in width; *Class V*: flat ridge form with inadequate height and width; *Class VI*: depressed ridge form with evident basal bone loss.[18] See also: *Cawood and Howell classification*.

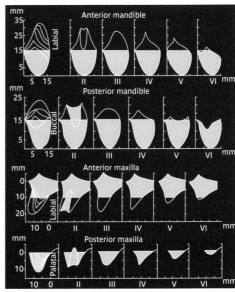

Classification of alveolar ridge morphology.
(Redrawn from Cawood and Howell[18] with permission.)

Radiographic assessment of a. r. Radiographic analysis of existing alveolar ridge dimensions using individual periapical radiographs, orthopantomogram, computer tomography, and/or digital volume tomography prior to implant placement to determine local bone anatomy, local pathology, and vital anatomic structures in close proximity.

Alveolar ridge augmentation Surgical augmentation of the alveolar ridge in a horizontal and/or vertical direction using one of several approaches based on the size and/or location of the defect.

    Bone grafting for a. r. a. Surgical procedure by which the residual alveolar ridge is enhanced in height and/or width with an autogenous graft, allograft, synthetic graft, or any combination of these materials.

    Calvarial bone grafting for a. r. a. Outer cortex of the calvarium is harvested for onlay alveolar ridge augmentation in patients with severe maxillary or mandibular atrophy; multiple blocks may be harvested. The bone is cortical in structure and tends to resorb less than iliac crest bone.[19]

A. r. a. in esthetic zone site   Requires not only the generation of sufficient volume for implant placement but also labial volume to mimic the natural contour of the alveolar process and support of the soft tissues. Attention also needs to be given to the coronal-apical level of the augmented bone and subsequently to the gingival margins so that an esthetic harmony among all maxillary anterior teeth is achieved and/or preserved.[20]

Guided bone regeneration for a. r. a.   Principle of guided bone regeneration (GBR) using barrier membranes, either resorbable or nonresorbable, to exclude certain cell types such as rapidly proliferating epithelium and connective tissue, thus promoting the growth of slower-growing cells capable of forming bone. GBR is often combined with bone grafting procedures.

Iliac bone grafting for a. r. a.   Common extraoral corticocancellous source of autogenous bone graft in cases where large block volumes are required for alveolar ridge augmentation. Two approaches to the iliac crest exist. Bone harvested from the anterior iliac crest, as described by Kalk et al[21], allows simultaneous surgery in the oral cavity. Harvesting from the posterior iliac crest, as described by Bloomquist and Feldman[22], requires that the patient be rotated in a prone position with a sandbag placed under the anterior iliac crest to support the pelvis, thus precluding simultaneous oral surgical access. The advantage of a posterior approach is that more than twice as much bone can be harvested, and postoperative morbidity is much less than that for the anterior approach. Block grafts may be combined with iliac crest particulate, which is harvested simultaneously.

Disadvantages of iliac crest harvesting include the need for general anesthesia, increased donor site morbidity, and potential for greater postoperative resorption rate as compared to intraoral sources of bone.[21-24]   See also: *Iliac crest*.

Le Fort I downfracture for a. r. a.   Surgical augmentation in a severely resorbed maxilla by a combination of a Le Fort I osteotomy and interposition of a bone graft harvested from a separate donor site within the patient (eg, iliac crest).[25]

Osteotome technique for a. r. a.
See: *Osteotome technique.*

Ramus bone grafting for a. r. a.
See: *Bone mill; Mandibular block graft, from the ramus.*

Split-ridge technique for a. r. a.   Augmentation procedure to increase the width of a narrow residual alveolar ridge by surgically splitting it or by expanding it with a series of osteotomes of increasing diameter. The procedure can be combined with simultaneous implant placement.

Titanium mesh – autogenous bone grafting for a. r. a.   Rarely performed augmentation procedure in which autogenous block and/or particulate grafts are covered by a titanium mesh fixed to the alveolar process with screws. While the graft is extremely stable, later removal of the titanium mesh device could cause adverse outcomes.[26]

Alveolar ridge defect   Circumscribed absence of tissue in a residual alveolar ridge.

Implant placement in a. r. d.   Requires simultaneous guided bone regeneration (GBR). Prerequisites for a simultaneous approach are: *(1)* implant placement in a correct prosthetic position, *(2)* good primary stability of the placed implant, and *(3)* an appropriate defect morphology that allows for a predictable regenerative treatment outcome. Vertical defects are more demanding than horizontal defects, as are one-wall, two-wall, and three-wall defects.

Morphology of a. r. d.   Classified as horizontal and/or vertical deficiencies. Classification is important for determining the prognosis of bone augmentation procedures. Clinicians tend to differentiate between one-wall, two-wall, and three-wall defects, similar to periodontal intrabony defects.

Alveolar ridge preservation
See: *Bio-Col technique.*

Alveolectomy   Surgical removal of parts of the alveolar process in the maxilla or mandible.

Alveoloplasty   Contouring of the alveolar process.

Alveolus   Socket of the alveolar process in which the tooth is attached by the periodontal ligament.

Amoxicillin   Semisynthetic derivative of ampicillin effective against a broad spectrum of gram-positive and gram-negative bacteria. This antibiotic is often used in the treatment of infections caused by susceptible strains of *Haemophilus influenzae, Escherichia coli, Proteus mirabilis, Neisseria gonorrhoeae, streptococci (*including *Streptococcus faecalis* and *S pneumoniae), and nonpenicillinase-producing staphylococci* of the oral cavity.[27]

Analog/analogue   Prosthetic component or element, the working surface of which is an exact duplicate of a specific surgical and/or prosthetic component. This element is typically incorporated in dental laboratory procedures to facilitate fabrication of an accurate master cast and/or prosthesis and can be incorporated into a model for patient education[28]   See also: *Replica.*

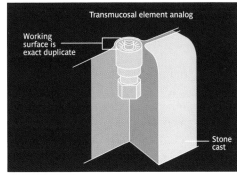

Analog/analogue.
(Redrawn from Yanase and Preston[28] with permission.)

Analysis of variance (ANOVA)   Statistical test to compare three or more groups on the mean value of a continuous response variable.[29]

Anatomic healing abutment   Prosthetic implant component that may be cylindrical in cross section but widens in diameter toward the coronal surface. The three-dimensional design of a healing abutment is intended to guide healing of the peri-implant sulcus for a cross-sectional shape that simulates a soft tissue emergence profile.

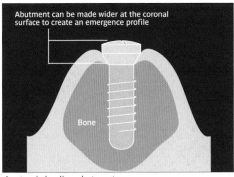

Anatomic healing abutment.

Anchorage, bicortical implant
See: *Bicortical stabilization.*

Anesthesia   Loss of sensation when an anesthetic drug is injected or topically applied to a particular area of the body. Local infiltration involves the application of an anesthetic agent to a localized area, whereas a nerve block will affect a particular region.

Angiogenesis Development of blood vessels in the embryo or any formation of new blood vessels. (See figure below.)

Angle, Bennett See: *Bennett movement.*

Angled/angulated abutment Prosthetic implant component designed to change direction from parallel along the long axis of the implant to a specified angle from parallel.

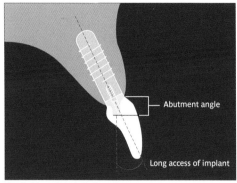

Angled/angulated abutment.

Angled/angulated implant Relative position of an implant to other adjacent implants or natural dentition.

Animal model Use of animals in biomedical research for conducting experiments. The quality, species, and breeding of the animal can help establish the type of animal to be used in the experiment.[31]

Anisotropic implant surface Implant surface that is not isotropic and may have different characteristics when measured or loaded in different directions.

Ankylosis Union or fusion between two joint components or between a tooth and the alveolar bone, often resulting from traumatic destruction of the periodontal membrane. When ankylosis is established, the tooth will gradually be replaced by bone-replacement resorption. See also: *Functional ankylosis.*

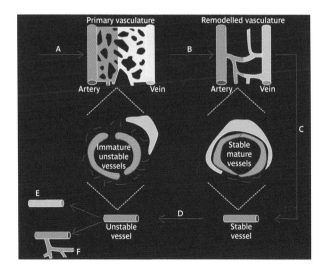

Angiogenesis.
(Redrawn from Yancopoulos et al[30] with permission.)

A

Anodization   Electrolytic treatment of a metallic surface, imparting an oxidized surface. Dye may be used to create a colored surface. Anodization in the manufacture of implant components facilitates color coding and/or recognition.

Anodizing surface treatment   Surfaces of various implant-related components (eg, abutments, screws) may be anodized to produce coloration, which assists with recognition by the clinician. Anodizing titanium with a yellow or golden color is thought to reduce the tendency for gray show-through of abutments when placed beneath thin tissues.   See also: *Anodization*.

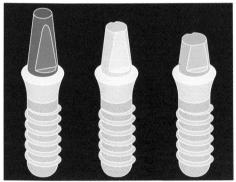

Anodizing surface treatment.

ANOVA   Abbreviation for *Analysis of variance*.

Anterior   Indication of a forward location also known as *front*. In oral anatomy, the anterior region of the mouth includes the jaw sections containing the incisors and canines.[32]

Anterior loop   Anatomic phenomenon of the mental nerve that is a continuation of an anterior loop beyond the mental foramen. Attention should be paid to this potential anatomic variation during implant treatment planning. Often anterior loops cannot be identified by radiographic examination. A distance of 4 mm anterior to the mental foramen has been recommended.[33]

Anterior nasal spine   Triangular protuberance of bone extending anteriorly from the inferior aspect of the nasal cavity at the midline, serving as an attachment point for the nasal cartilage. This bony structure is often used as an intraoral source of autogenous bone for grafting procedures of smaller volumes.

Anteroposterior spread (AP spread)   Distance from a line drawn between the posterior edges of the two most distal implants in an arch and the midpoint of the most anterior implant in the arch. This measurement is used to calculate the maximum posterior cantilever length of the prosthesis, which is usually 1.5 times the AP spread.

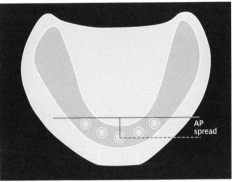

Anteroposterior spread (AP spread).

Antibiotic   Substance, such as penicillin, produced by fungi, bacteria, or other organisms that can inhibit or destroy the growth of other microorganisms. Antibiotics are widely used in the prevention and treatment of infectious diseases.[34]   See also: *Amoxicillin; Penicillin.*

Antibiotic prophylaxis   Prescribed for patients pre- or peri-operatively to prevent postsurgical infections. Widely used with different regimens, although no consensus exists for use in routine procedures. Clinicians may routinely use it in patients with large – volume augmentations (eg, block grafting, sinus augmentation) or in patients (such as diabetics) with compromised wound healing. In patients with a risk of endocarditis, a standard regimen has been established and is recommended for certain types of dental procedures.[35]

Antirotation   Resistance to rotation or ability of implant stack components to resist loosening.   See also: *Stack*.

Antral floor   Inferior bony wall of the maxillary sinus cavity.

Antral floor grafting
See: *Maxillary sinus floor elevation*.

Antral mucosa
See: *Maxillary sinus membrane*.

Antrostomy   Surgically created opening into the antrum.[36]

Antrum   Cavity or chamber in the body, often within bone. Maxillary antrum refers to the maxillary sinus.   See also: *Maxillary sinus*.

Antrum of Highmore   See: *Maxillary sinus*.

AP spread   Abbreviation for *Anteroposterior spread*.

Apex   Anatomic end of a tooth root or root-form implant.[10]

Apical   Referring to, or in the direction of, a root apex.   See also: *Apex*.

Apical offset   Design feature at the apical portion of an implant that allows for expansion, resulting in circumferential offset and an increase in the overall diameter of the implant at the apical portion.[37]

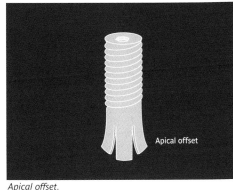

Apical offset.

Apically positioned flap
See: *Flap, apically positioned*.

Aplasia   Incomplete development of an organ or tissue. Congenital absence may be characteristic.

Apoptosis   Morphologic pattern of cell death affecting single cells and marked by shrinkage of the cell, condensation of chromatin, formation of cytoplasmic blebs, and fragmentation of the cell into membrane-bound apoptotic bodies that are eliminated by phagocytosis.

Appositional bone growth   See: *Bone modeling*.

Arch   Bony arc formed by the maxillary or the mandibular teeth or residual ridge when viewed occlusally.[38]

Archwire   Wire attached to two or more teeth or implants, generally used to guide or retain teeth during orthodontic therapy.

Arm prosthesis   Artificial replacement for part or all of the human arm.   See also: *Somatoprosthesis*.

Artery Blood vessel that carries oxygenated blood from the heart to tissues and organs.

Articulating tape Ink-impregnated paper or silk ribbon used to identify contacting occlusal or incisal surfaces.[10]

Articulation Static and dynamic relationships of contacting occlusal surfaces during function. It also pertains to the junctions or contacting surfaces of bones of the skeleton. See also: *Canine-protected articulation*.

Articulator Apparatus designed to mechanically orient the essential elements of mastication (ie, temporomandibular joints, jaws, and teeth) in their simulated spatial relationship outside the mouth. The design is based on the degree of mandibular movement simulation desired for the development of an occlusal scheme.[10]

Fully adjustable a. Articulating instrument permitting the simulation of three-dimensional mandibular movement and capable of accepting three-dimensional jaw registration records.[39]

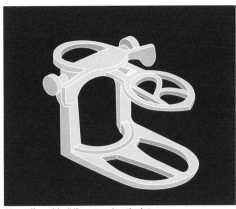

Nonadjustable (Hinge-type) articulator.
(Redrawn from Starcke and Engelmeier[40] with permission.)

Semi-adjustable a. Instrument capable of simulating vertical and horizontal movement with or without temporomandibular joint orientation. Joint articular references are commonly reversed with condylar guidance developed according to mechanical equivalents based on anatomic averages. Some semi-adjustable articulators provide for temporomandibular joint orientation and may be either Nonarcon (condylar elements in the upper member) or Arcon (condylar elements in the lower member as in the human situation).[39]

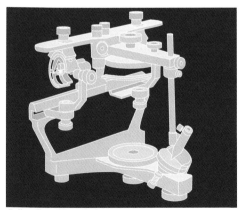

Fully adjustable articulator.

Nonadjustable a. Hinge-type instrument capable of retaining maxillary and mandibular jaw casts in an established vertical relationship while providing possible vertical motion in an arcing pattern.[39]

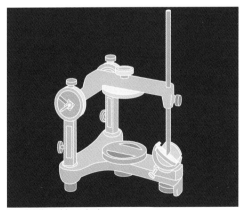

Semi-adjustable articulator.

Artificial limb Artificial replacement for part or all of a human arm or leg. See also: *Somatoprosthesis*.

Asepsis The state of being free of living pathogenic microorganisms; the process of removing pathogenic microorganisms; or protecting against infection by such organisms.[41]

Atherosclerosis Form of arteriosclerosis characterized by the deposition of atheromatous plaques containing cholesterol and lipids on the innermost layer of the walls of large- and medium-sized arteries.[42]

Atresia Absence or closure of a natural body passage. May also refer to loss of a body part through degeneration.[43] See also: *Congenital atresia.*

Atrophic Reduced both in volume and substance. Bone loss in volume can be a reduction both in width and height, and loss of substance can mean reduction in thickness of cortical bone and width and number of trabeculae.

Atrophic alveolar bone Alveolar bone characterized by resorption after tooth removal. When functional stimulus disappears, the alveolar bone will atrophy.

Atrophy Wasting away or decrease in the size of an organ or tissue, as from death and subsequent reabsorption of cells, diminished cellular proliferation, pressure, ischemia, malnutrition, decreased function, or hormonal changes.[44] See also: *Alveolar atrophy; Residual ridge resorption.*

Attached gingiva Portion of gingiva that is firm, dense, stippled, and tightly bound to underlying periosteum and tooth.[45]

Attachment Element incorporated into the design of a prosthesis to aid in the retention and/or stabilization of the prosthesis. The retention design can be classified as mechanical, frictional fit, and/or magnetic. Comprised of two parts, the matrix is the receptacle component, and the corresponding patrix closely fits within the matrix either mechanically or

with a frictional fit.[46,47] See also: *Gold cylinder attachment; Magnetic attachment; Nonrotating gold cylinder.*

Connective tissue a.
 See: *Connective tissue attachment.*

Attachment element Part of the prosthetic component made as a separate unit fitting onto the transmucosal element. "If there is no separate attachment element, the restoration is part of and fabricated with the retentive element." It is the element onto which the restoration is fabricated as cast-to, cemented, or screwed into position.[48]

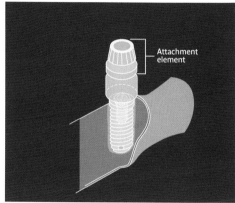

Attachment element.
(Redrawn from Yanase and Preston[48] with permission.)

Attachment level Relative distance from a fixed reference point on a tooth or dental implant to the tip of the periodontal probe during soft tissue diagnostic probing. Health of the attachment apparatus can affect the measurement. See also: *Clinical attachment level.*

Attachment screw Element directly relating to the specific prosthetic component to which it attaches. Typically, the prosthetic component is seated, and the attachment screw is threaded through the prosthetic component into another component in the implant system, such as the implant. It can be manufactured of various materials, such as gold alloy or titanium.[49,50] (See figure next page.)

A

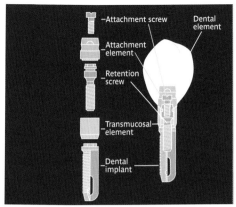

Attachment screw.
(Redrawn from Yanase and Preston[49] with permission.)

Attachment system Design of a particular type of retentive mechanism employing compatible matrix and patrix corresponding components. *Matrix* refers to the receptacle component of the attachment system, and *patrix* refers to the portion that has a frictional fit and engages the matrix. Corresponding components are passive once engaged and offer resistance to displacement either through a direct mechanical mechanism or a frictional fit. See also: *Adjustable attachment system; Ball attachment system; Bar attachment system; Magnet attachment system; Telescopic coping attachment system.*

Augmentation Grafting procedure designed to increase the volume of existing tissues, usually referring to bone for the purpose of adequate bony support around implants and/or improving tissue contours for esthetic purposes.

Auricular prosthesis Fixed/removable artificial replacement for all or part of a human ear.[10,32]

Autocrine Transfer of chemical compounds as hormones and growth factors within the cell.

Autogenous bone graft Bone graft taken from an intraoral or extraoral site and placed in the same individual. Origin of the graft will determine whether it is cortical, corticocancellous, or cancellous in nature. Particulate grafts may be harvested with hand instruments or prepared by introducing chips into a bone mill. Block grafts can be harvested when a cortical component exists (ie, symphysis, ramus buccal shelf, calvarium, or iliac crest), when volume is not sufficient, and/or if the need to retard resorption is required. Autogenous bone grafts are often mixed with allografts, alloplasts, or xenografts. Called also *autograft*. See also: *Alveolar ridge augmentation; Bone graft.*

Autogenous graft Tissue transferred from one location to another within the same individual. See also: *Autogenous bone graft; Bone graft; Soft tissue augmentation.*

Autograft See: *Autogenous bone graft.*

Autologous bone See: *Autogenous bone graft.*

Autopolymerizing resin Resin capable of polymerization via a chemical activator and catalyzing agent. Called also *cold-* or *self-curing resin.*

Avascular Lacking in blood supply or vasculature.

Axial loading Application of load, usually by the forces of occlusion, in the direction of the long axis of an implant body or tooth. Compare: *Nonaxial Loading.*

B

Backscattered electron (BSE) imaging High-resolution imaging of a surface using electronics, similar to how a light microscope uses visible light. The advantages of BSE over light microscopy include greater magnification and much greater depth of field. This method is most commonly performed via application of accelerating voltages of 10 kV or more to the specimen while detecting high-energy electrons that backscatter quasi-elastically off the sample. For imaging of surface detail, the application of a lower-accelerating voltage results in less beam penetration, spread, and overall specimen damage.

Bacterial collagenase Any of various collagenases purified from a variety of microbes; they preferentially cleave collagen on the N-terminal side of glycine residues and occur in several classes of differing specificity. Bacterial collagenases are used in tissue disruption for cell harvesting.

Bacterial leakage Colonization and release of bacteria at the interface of an oral implant abutment and implant.[1]

Bacterium (pl: *bacteria*) Member of a group of ubiquitous, single-celled microorganisms that have a prokaryotic (primitive) cell type. Many of these are etiologic in diseases that affect all life forms, including humans and other animals. See also: *Actinobacillus actinomycetemcomitans; Fusobacterium nucleatum.*

BAHA Abbreviation for *Bone-anchored hearing aid.*

Balanced occlusion Existing or developed simultaneous harmonious occlusal contact of the teeth throughout the dental arch during mandibular centric and eccentric movements; especially important for removable complete dentures to achieve stability during function.[2,3] See also: *Articulation.*

Ball attachment system Specific design of a mechanical attachment in which the patrix fits into the matrix in a ball-and-socket type of relation. Each element is incorporated into either the natural tooth as part of a restoration or as an abutment on the implant with the reciprocal element incorporated into the prosthesis. The patrix, or ball, can be made of plastic or metal alloy of various diameters and with varied amounts of resistance.[4]

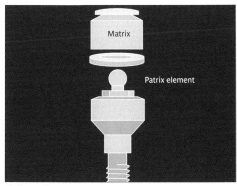

Ball attachment system.

Bar Round, half-round, or elliptically shaped metallic segment with greater length than width. A bar is commonly used to connect components of a prosthesis such as abutments, crowns, or parts of a removable partial denture. It also can be used to provide support, stability, and/or retention for a prosthesis.[2,3]   See also: *Dolder bar; Hader bar*.

Bar attachment system   Specific design of an attachment in which the patrix spans a specified width that the matrix matches. Each element is part of a prosthetic structure that spans two or more natural teeth and/or implants and is fixed intraorally with the matrix, which is incorporated within the prosthesis. Once the components are engaged by riders, clips, or microplungers, there is resistance to displacement through either a mechanical mechanism or frictional fit. [5]

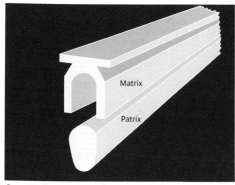

Bar attachment system (in cross section).

Four implants with b. a. s.   Mechanical attachment incorporated into and fabricated as part of a prosthesis mesostructure supported by four implants.

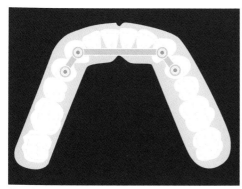

Four implants with bar attachment system.

Two-implant overdenture with b. a. s.   Mechanical attachment incorporated into and fabricated as part of a prosthesis mesostructure supported by two implants.

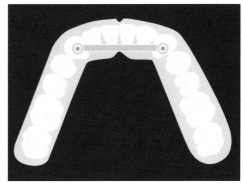

Two-implant overdenture with bar attachment system.

Bar clip retention   See: *Clip bar overdenture; Retainer; Retention*.

Bar overdenture (implant)   See: *Clip bar overdenture*.

Bar splint   Connecting bar for adding rigidity and/or stability between teeth or implants. It is also used to fixate displaced or movable body parts as a result of trauma or surgery.[2] See also: *Splinting*.

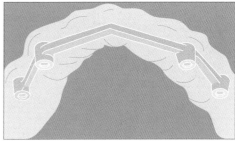

Bar splint.

Barium sulfate   Alkaline earth metal ($BaSO_4$). *Barium* is derived from the Greek word *barys*, meaning *heavy* and is generally a toxic substance in water-soluble compounds. Barium sulfate, however, is insoluble in water, and because it is even insoluble in hydrochloric acid, it can be used as a medical contrast medium to examine the gastrointestinal tract.

Barrier membrane   Used in guided bone regeneration (GBR) to locally augment deficient sites in implant patients. By creating a secluded space, the barrier prevents epithelial cells and fibroblasts from proliferating into the augmentation site, whereas the slower-growing angiogenic and osteogenic cells have exclusive access to the membrane-protected space. The first membranes were made of bio-inert expanded polytetrafluoroethylene (e-PTFE), which is nonresorbable and therefore required removal with a second surgical procedure. Bioresorbable membranes, either of synthetic polymers or of animal-derived collagen, are often preferred in daily practice. Although their barrier function is limited in time, they do not require a second surgical procedure for membrane removal. Barrier membranes exclude undesirable cell types from entering the secluded area of the bony or periodontal defect during healing. Membrane configurations are designed for specific applications; vary in shape, size, and thickness.   See also: *Guided bone regeneration (GBR); Guided tissue regeneration (GTR); Collagen membrane; Expanded polytetrafluoroethylene (e-PTFE) membrane.*

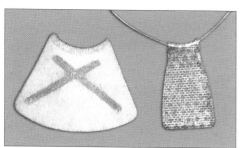

Barrier membranes specially designed for treatment of recession defects. (left Nonresorbable titanium-reinforced expanded polytetrafluoroethylene (e – PTFE) membrane; right Bioresorbable polylactic acid and citric acid ester-based membrane.)
(Reprinted from Lindhe et al[6] with permission.)

Basal bone   Supporting bone in the mandible that underlies and is continuous with the alveolar process and houses the major nerves and vessels. It also functions as a site of muscle attachment and is resistant to resorption.[7]

Basic fibroblast growth factor (bFGF)
   See: *Fibroblast growth factor (FGF).*

Basic multicellular unit (BMU)   Fully developed cortical bone remodeling unit comprising an elongated cylindrical structure about 2 mm long and 0.2 mm wide, which travels through bone in a controlled direction. The BMU preserves its size, shape, and internal organization for many months. Maintenance of this unique entity requires continued recruitment of new osteoclasts and osteoblasts in appropriate numbers and the growth of new blood vessels, nerves, and connective tissue. The end result of each new BMU is one new Haversian system or osteon.

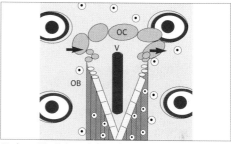

Basic multicellular unit (BMU).
A BMU contains osteoclasts OC, as well as vascular structures V and osteoblasts OB.
(Redrawn from Lang et al[6] with permission.)

B cell   White blood cell derived from bone marrow. As part of the immune system, B cells (or *bursa-equivalent cells*) may differentiate and become antibody-producing plasma cells. Called also *B lymphocyte.*

Bending moment   Rotary effect of a force potentially causing deformation through torque.

Bennett movement   Translatory or bodily side shift of the mandible that occurs with lateral mandibular movement. During lateral mandibular movement, as the advancing condyle path intersects with the sagittal plane, an angle known as the *Bennett angle* is formed.[3] (See figure next page)

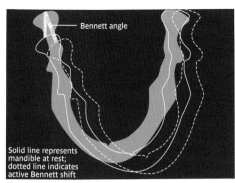

Bennett movement.
(Redrawn from Sharry[9] with permission.)

Beveled incision   Technique by which incisions are made at an acute angle (less than 90 degrees) to the gingival or mucosal surface, rather than perpendicularly.

bFGF   Abbreviation for *Basic fibroblast growth factor*.   See: *Fibroblast growth factor (FGF)*.

BIC   Abbreviation for *Bone-implant contact*.

Bicortical implant anchorage
See: *Bicortical stabilization*.

Bicortical stabilization   Practice of engaging both the superior and inferior cortices of bone at the time of implant placement. For an edentulous anterior mandible, the tip of the implant engages the inferior cortex while the neck of the implant engages the superior cortex to maximize initial stability of the implant.

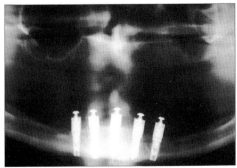

Bicortical stabilization. (Courtesy of T. D. Taylor.)

Bidirectional crest distraction   Distraction approach designed to overcome the inherent difficulty in controlling the distraction vector in conventional, unidirectional devices. An additional inclination rod allows for buccal-oral (lingual) distraction in addition to vertical distraction.[10]

Bilateral stabilization
See: *Cross-arch stabilization*.

Bioabsorbable material   Solid polymeric material that can dissolve in body fluids without any change of the polymer or decrease in molecular mass.

Bioactive glass   Ceramic material that stimulates or otherwise promotes biologic activity. It consists of silicophosphate chains that bond ionically to compounds such as CaO, CaF_2, Na_2O, ZnO, TiO_2 and NiO, among others. It may undergo ionic translocations in vivo, or exchange ions or molecular groups in an osseous recipient site, and thereby osseointegrate. Bioactive glass may be resorbable and is useful as a delivery system in bone engineering.   See also: *Ceramic*.

Bioactivity   Effect of implant material that allows interaction and bond formation with living tissues. Implant bioactivity may depend upon material composition, topography, and chemical or physical surface variations.

Bioadhesion   Result of a process whereby a chemical attachment between biologic and other materials is obtained.

Bio-Col technique   Technique developed to preserve the ridge in the esthetic zone. A tooth is extracted via a low-trauma technique to maintain intact bony walls and surrounding gingival anatomy without flap reflection. The extraction socket is grafted up to the alveolar crest with an anorganic bovine bone substitute, covered with a collagen plug, and sutured in place with a horizontal mattress suture. A removable or fixed provisional restoration with an ovate pontic extending 3 to 4 mm subgingivally is placed, compressing the collagen plug and supporting the surrounding soft tissue. This technique has also been described in combination with immediate implant placement and with a buccal defect, whereby the defect is first lined with a collagen membrane.[11]

Biocompatibility Condition whereby the body does not respond to a foreign substance (eg, metal) but recognizes it immunologically as self. Biocompatible materials do not lead to acute or chronic inflammatory responses nor do they prevent proper differentiation of implant-surrounding tissues.

Biocompatible Capable of existing together; acceptable to the body. This term is used to describe blood, organs, or tissue that can be transplanted or transfused into a patient's body without being rejected. It describes a biodynamic process in which a material neither elicits an immune response nor is rejected by the host.[12,13]

Biodegradable material Solid polymeric material that breaks down because of macromolecular degradation with dispersion in vivo; no proof for elimination from the body.

Bioengineering Use of engineering in biomedical technology such as the movement analysis of body parts or prostheses. See also: *Tissue engineering.*

Bioerodible material Solid polymeric material that shows surface degradation and resorbs in vivo; reflects total elimination of the foreign material.

Biofilm Thin layer of microorganisms adhering to the surface of a structure, organic or inorganic, together with the polymers that they secrete. See also: *Plaque.*

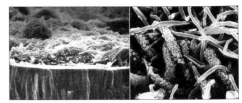

Biofilm (scanning electron micrograph; high magnification). (Courtesy of C. M. Cobb.)

Bioglass See: *Bioactive glass.*

Bioinert Describes a biomaterial that does not elicit a biologic response or is unaffected by the adjacent biologic environment.

Biointegration See: *Osseointegration.*

Biologic width Structure of the attachment apparatus containing connective tissue attachment, junctional epithelium, and gingival sulcus.

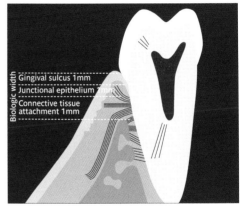

Gingival sulcus 1mm
Junctional epithelium 1mm
Connective tissue attachment 1mm

Biologic width.
(Reprinted from Nevins[14] with permission.)

Normal b. w. Measures 1 mm for each structure, including the connective tissue attachment, junctional epithelium, and gingival sulcus.

Biomaterial Nonviable material used as a medical device, intended to interact with biologic systems. See also: *Bioactive glass; Titanium (Ti).*

Biomechanical load model   Simulation or model of load pattern in and adjacent to a structure.   See also: *Biomechanics*.

Biomechanical test   Examination of biologic tissues, systems, and artificial materials within biologic systems through mechanical means.

Biomechanics   Application of mechanical principles and design to biologic structures; the interface between biology and mechanics.

Biomimetics   Science of reconstructing or mimicking natural processes with the expectation that regeneration will follow.   See also: *Tissue engineering*.

Biomineralization   Formation or accumulation of minerals into biologic tissues such as bone and teeth. The process of biologic mineralization is not completely understood. Interstitial fluids are supersaturated with mineral hydroxyapatite, and calcium binding proteins such as osteocalcin are deposited and may play a role in the formation of crystal nuclei.[15,16]

Bio-Oss
See: *Bovine-derived anorganic bone matrix*.

Biopsy   See: *Bone biopsy*.

Bioresorbable   The capacity to become lysed or assimilated in vivo.

Bioresorbable material   Solid polymeric material that shows bulk degradation and further resorbs in vivo, resulting in total elimination of the initial foreign material.   Compare: *Resorbable*.

Bio-stimulating laser
See: *Low-level laser therapy*.

Bisphosphonate   Pyrophosphate analog that blocks osteoclastic activity by interfering with the function of guanosine triphosphate bind-

ing proteins, thereby leading to osteoclastic apoptosis. Therapeutic treatment of diseases such as osteoporosis and Paget disease rely on oral bisphosphonates to inhibit osteoclastic function.   See also: *Osteonecrosis*.

Biting force   Force generated by contraction of elevator muscles of mandible acting against the maxilla.

Black space   See: *Black triangle*.

Black triangle   Missing papilla between teeth when the interproximal bone has been reduced in height. The coronal-apical distance between the bone crest level and the contact point of adjacent teeth will determine if a papilla can be consistently maintained. A similar relationship has been shown for single-tooth implants. It has been proposed that the distance between two adjacent implants is also important for the maintenance of interproximal bone height, which may then influence the height of interimplant papillae.[17-20]

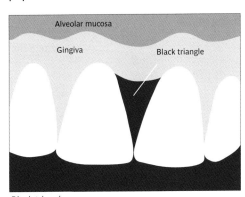

Black triangle.

Blade   Flat instrument with one or more sharp edges used for cutting.[21]

Blade implant   Design-specific type of implant that is categorized as an endosteal implant. Blade implants can vary in width and length and are intended to be placed within bone as a one-piece implant. Both the implant that is the endosteal portion and the transmucosal component that serves as an abutment intra-orally are included.[22-24]

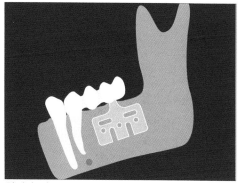
Blade implant.

Blanching   Process by which soft tissues become pale or cyanotic with pressure. The redness of erythema decreases and then returns when pressure is applied and released.

Bleeding   Condition involving the loss of blood internally (when blood leaks from blood vessels inside the body); externally through a natural opening (such as the oral cavity); or externally through a break in the skin.

Bleeding on probing   Process of bleeding from the gingival sulcus or periodontal pocket following standard measurement by periodontal probe.

Block bone graft   Includes blocks harvested either from the mandibular symphysis or ramus buccal shelf that are used for localized ridge augmentation procedures.[25-27]   See also: *Alveolar ridge augmentation; Bone graft*.

Blood cell   Element found in peripheral blood. In humans the normal mature form is a non-nucleated, yellowish, biconcave disk, adapted by virtue of its configuration and its hemoglobin content to the transport of oxygen.   See also: *Erythrocyte*.

Blood clot   Semisolidified mass in the bloodstream formed of an aggregation of blood factors, primarily platelets and fibrin, with entrapment of cellular elements. Called also *coagulum*.

Blood platelet   See: *Platelet*.

B lymphocyte   See: *B cell*.

BMD   Abbreviation for *Bone mineral density*.

BMP   Abbreviation for *Bone morphogenetic protein*.

BMPR   Abbreviation for *Bone morphogenetic protein receptors*.

BMU   Abbreviation for *Basic multicellular unit*.

Bone   Highest achievement in the evolution of supporting tissues. Mineralized collagen with enclosed cells, where formation of intercellular connections via cytoplasmic processes allow for transport of metabolites from surfaces (lining cells) to deeper osteocytes. Excellent mechanical behavior and a unique potential for regeneration.   See also: *Alveolar bone; Atrophic alveolar bone; Basal bone; Bundle bone; Cancellous bone; Cortical bone; Corticocancellous bone; Lamellar bone; Parallel-fibered bone; Trabecular bone; Woven bone*.

Bone-anchored hearing aid (BAHA)   Electronic device affixed to the temporal bone in the peri-auricular area with skin-penetrating implant abutments for the amplification of sound in hearing-impaired patients.[28,29] (See figure next page.)

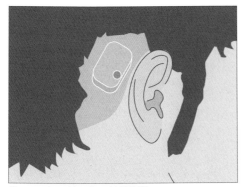

Bone-anchored hearing aid (BAHA).

Bone augmentation
See: *Alveolar ridge augmentation.*

Bone biopsy   Bone taken from a suspected area of pathology for diagnostic purposes.

Bone cell   Bone cells include osteoblasts, which are responsible for bone formation, and osteoclasts, which are responsible for bone resorption. The osteoblasts originate from mesenchymal stem cells, whereas the osteoclasts (giant cells) belong to the hematopoietic system with granulocyte – macrophage progenitor cells as their precursors. The osteoblasts become osteocytes and lining cells after a period of formative function. The osteoclasts may disintegrate into mononuclear cells or undergo apoptosis after function.   See also: *Lining cells; Osteoblast; Osteoclast; Osteocyte.*

Bone conduction   See: *Osteoconduction.*

Bone curettage   Removal of soft tissue either from a bony surface by scraping with a curette in preparation for implant placement and/or alveolar ridge augmentation, or from a bony cavity following the removal of pathology.

Bone derivative   Left common denominator for bone substitutes developed via chemical extraction processes.

Bone expansion   See: *Alveolar ridge augmentation, Split-ridge technique for.*

Bone fibers   See: *Sharpey connective tissue fibers.*

Bone fill   Clinical restoration of bone tissue in a treated osseous defect. It addresses neither the presence nor absence of histologic evidence of new connective tissue attachment nor the formation of a new periodontal ligament in the case of tooth-supporting bone. Measurement can be accomplished radiographically, clinically (by re-entry), or histologically.

Bone fracture   Break in bone, usually the result of trauma. It can also be caused by an acquired disease of bone or by abnormal formation associated with bone disease. Fractures are further classified by their character and location: greenstick, spiral, comminuted, transverse, compound, and compression.

Bone graft   Bone taken from a donor site of the patient (autogenous) or from an outside source (allograft, alloplastic graft, or xenograft). A bone graft is used to augment a bone deficiency in the alveolar ridge. It can be used with simultaneous or subsequent implant placement.   See also: *Allogeneic bone graft; Alloplastic graft; Alveolar ridge augmentation; Autogenous bone graft; Onlay graft; Xenograft.*

Donor site for b. g.   Source of an autogenous bone graft may be intraoral or extraoral in origin. Intraoral sources include adjacent cortical bone, anterior nasal spine, retromolar area, maxillary tuberosity, ramus, buccal shelf, and the mandibular symphysis. Extraoral sources of bone grafts include cranium, iliac crest, and tibia. Depending on the source, the graft is either more cortical or more cancellous in nature.

Bone harvest Acquisition of bone from a patient for an autogenous graft, from deceased individuals for an allogeneic graft, or from animals for a xenograft. See also: *Cranial bone harvest; Iliac crest graft; Tibial bone harvest.*

Bone healing Cellular events, recapitulating embryogenesis. After initiation of woven bone formation, deposition of parallel-fibered bone ensues. These two primary types of bone repair the defect within weeks; thereafter, the formation of perivascularly arranged lamellar bone takes place with simultaneous resorption of the two primary bone types. This substitution, which gives strength to the bone, may take months to years, depending upon the size of defect. Finally, a structural rearrangement of trabeculae in response to function (Wolff law) takes place. Healing of fractures of long bones may often be characterized by a callus formation in the initial stages, where woven bone is mixed with cartilage, resulting in a clinically as well as radiologically visible thickening of the fracture site. This callus will disappear along with the osseous maturation.

Bone-implant contact (BIC) Direct contact of bone with the surface of an endosseous implant as seen microscopically. The ratio of bone contact to implant surface (percent) is used to evaluate implant surface topogra-

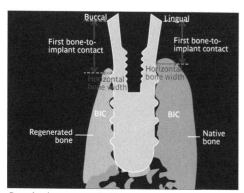

Bone-implant contact (BIC).
(*Reprinted from Von Arx et al[90] with permission.*)

phies and materials. See also: *Implant survival; Loading, Effects on bone-implant contact; Stress distribution.*

B

Bone-implant interface Line of demarcation between the nonliving surface of an endosseous implant and the living bone it contacts. Numerous factors may influence the degree to which bone heals in contact with the implant surface, including surface texture, surface contamination, time since placement, and extent of functional loading, among others. See also: *Implant interface.*

Immediate loading considerations for b.-i. i.
See: *Primary stability; Secondary stability.*

Implant design and b.-i. i. Architecture of the implant stack or its overall design, including thread design and pitch. It affects the ability of the implant to be placed into its osteotomy with primary stability and is deemed necessary for osseointegration to occur.

Micromotion and b.-i. i. Micromotion during initial osseointegration may precipitate failure of osseointegration to occur. See also: *Micromotion.*

Overload and b.-i. i. Generally assumed that occlusal overloading can result in failure at the bone-implant interface, although the limited scientific evidence does not support this assumption.[31-35] See also: *Occlusal overload.*

Bone induction Interaction among pluripotential cells and bone morphogenetic proteins (BMPs) that converts these cells to osteoblasts.

Bone loss Physiologic loss of bone mass. The peak of mineral density is reached between 30 and 40 years of age; women lose about 35% of cortical bone and 50% of trabecular bone, whereas men lose about two-thirds of these amounts. See also: *Osteoporosis*.

Bone marrow Apart from cells of the hematopoietic system, the marrow contains mesenchymal stem cells, osteoprogenitor cells, and osteoblasts. Additionally, elements of fat tissue and connective tissue are seen.

Bone mass Amount of bone, often estimated by absorptiometry, viewed as a volume minus the marrow cavity. Optimal balance in the composition of the bone is reached between 30 and 40 years of age. In this age period, the ratio between cortical and trabecular bone to bone marrow assures that maximum strength is reached by a minimum of bone mass.

Bone matrix Contains collagen type I (90%) and noncollagenous protein (about 10%): osteonectin, osteopontin, bone sialoprotein, and growth factors (cytokines) such as insulin-like growth factors (IGF1 and IGF2), transforming growth factor beta 1 (TGF-β1), platelet-derived growth factor (PDGF), acidic and basic fibroblast growth factors (aFGF and bFGF), and bone morphogenetic proteins (BMPs).

Bone mill Device used intraoperatively to particulate autogenous bone chips into smaller particles for localized alveolar ridge augmentation.

Bone mineral Mineral in bone composed of calcium carbonate (10%), calcium and magnesium fluoride (5%), and calcium phosphates (85%), present primarily as hydroxyapatite.

Bone mineral density (BMD) Density of bone expressed in cm^2, measured by dual-energy x-ray absorptiometry (DEXA).

Bone modeling Processes producing functionally purposeful skeletal organs aimed at characteristic adult shape and form; includes longitudinal, transversal, and appositional growth.

Bone morphogenetic protein (BMP) Special group of the transforming growth factor beta (TGF-β) superfamily of growth factors with the unique property of stimulating mesenchymal stem cells to differentiate toward a chondro- and osteoblastic lineage. BMP–2, BMP–3, and BMP–7 have proven to be powerful stimulators of bone healing. Several BMPs such as BMP–2, BMP–4, and BMP–7 are known to induce the expression of core-binding factor alpha 1 (CBFα1). See also: *Isoforms*.

Osteoinductive properties of b. m. p. The BMP family of proteins, most notably BMP–2, BMP–4, and BMP–7, are known to promote de novo bone formation through the process of osteoinduction. Bone may be formed with a cartilage intermediate stage, as in the situation of endochondral bone formation or directly, as in intramembranous bone formation.

Bone morphogenetic protein 2 (BMP–2) Polypeptide that belongs to the transforming growth factor beta (TGF-β) superfamily of proteins. Like other BMPs, it plays an important role in the development of bone and cartilage. It is involved in the Hedgehog pathway, TGF-β–signaling pathway, and cytokine-cytokine receptor interaction, as well as cardiac cell differentiation and epithelial to mesenchymal transition.

Bone morphogenetic protein 4 (BMP–4) Polypeptide belonging to the transforming growth factor beta (TGF-β) superfamily of proteins. Like other BMPs, it is involved in bone and cartilage development, specifically tooth and limb development and fracture repair, and has been shown to be involved in muscle development and bone mineralization.

B

Bone morphogenetic protein 5 (BMP – 5) Polypeptide member of the transforming growth factor beta (TGF-β) superfamily of proteins. BMP – 5 may play a role in certain cancers. Like other BMPs, BMP – 5 is inhibited by molecules chordin and noggin. It is expressed in the trabecular meshwork, lung, liver, and optic nerve, and may be involved in the development and normal function of these organs.

Bone morphogenetic protein 7 (BMP – 7) Member of the transforming growth factor beta (TGF-β) superfamily of proteins. Similar to other members of the BMP family of proteins, it plays a key role in the transformation of mesenchymal cells into bone and cartilage. It is inhibited by noggin. BMP – 7 may be involved in bone homeostasis and is expressed in the brain, kidneys, and bladder. BMP – 7 has been shown to induce SMAD – 1 as well as multiple biomarkers of osteoblast differentiation. Called also *Osteogenic protein 1*.

Bone morphogenetic protein receptors (BM-PR) Transmembrane receptors that are present in a wide variety of cells and mediate BMP signals. They comprise serine or threonine kinase receptors composed of subtypes I and II.

Bone necrosis See: *Osteonecrosis*.

Bone-plate device with external activation screws See: *Alveolar distraction osteogenesis.*

Bone preparation Act of readying the bony site for implant, transplant, or graft placement. To achieve implant osseointegration, a low-trauma preparation of the implant bed is prerequisite. Bone preparation with several drills of increasing diameter is performed using copious saline solution to provide cooling.

Bone quality See: *Alveolar bone, Quality of.*

Bone quantity See: *Alveolar bone, Quantity of.*

Bone regeneration Renewal or repair of lost bone tissue. Also: Cellular events during wound healing; recapitulation of cellular events of embryogenesis. The quantitative extent is defect dependent and influenced by cellular race. See also: *Bone remodeling; Bone morphogenetic protein (BMP); Bone scaffold; Gene therapy; Growth factor; Guided bone regeneration (GBR); Periodontal bone regeneration.*

Bone regeneration strategies Use of polypeptide growth factors to serve as mediators to promote osteoblast migration, mitogenesis, or matrix synthesis leading to bone regeneration. See also: *Growth factor*.

Bone remodeling Basic physiologic remodeling of bone takes place in a biologically coupled system of activation, resorption, formation (ARF). Histomorphologically, the process starts in cortical bone as a cutting cone, consisting of a group of osteoclasts, digs a tunnel with a breakdown of 20 µm per day with a simultaneous increase in diameter of the tunnel in magnitude of 5 µm per day until a width of approximately 100 µm in radius is reached. When the resorption ceases, the osteoclasts are replaced by osteoblasts after a short resting period. The osteoblasts form new lamellar bone at a speed of 1 µm per day, and thereby the tunnel is closed again. The length of the entire cone is typically around 1,500 to 1,600 µm. The entire course is also named *creeping substitution*. Similar remodeling takes place in trabecular bone as surface resorption, creating a 60- to 70-µm – deep crateriform cavity that is filled in with lamellar osteoid over a 4-month period. See also: *Basic multicellular unit (BMU); Bone remodeling unit (BRU); Bone structural unit (BSU).* (See figure next page.)

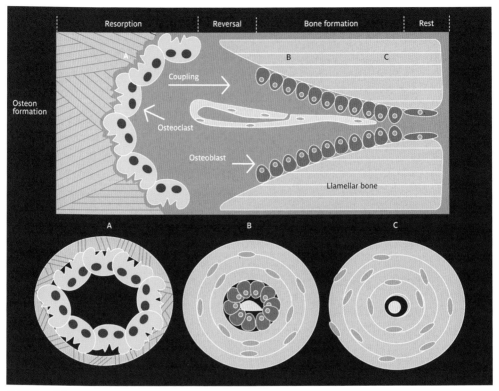

Bone remodeling.
(Redrawn from Buser et al[36] with permission.)

Bone remodeling unit (BRU) Group of osteoblasts and osteoclasts involved in the process of bone remodeling. See also: *Bone remodeling.*

Bone scaffold Process of bone formation that occurs through the utilization of a scaffolding matrix that may deliver cells, genes, or proteins. The scaffold may be osteoinductive or osteoconductive and serves to maintain the architecture of the anatomic defect.

Bone sounding Simple preoperative procedure performed under local anesthesia using a fine needle with a rubber stopper. The needle is used to penetrate soft tissues to assess the form and volume of the existing alveolar ridge.

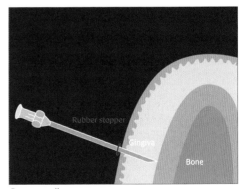

Bone sounding.

Bone spreader See: *Alveolar ridge augmentation, Split-ridge technique for; Osteotome.*

Bone stimulation Initiation of bone formation around endosseous implants by pulsed electromagnetic fields. Must be performed within very early stages of healing, ie, during the first and second weeks; after 2 weeks, no effect can be measured. This principle has only been used in animal studies.[37]

Bone strength Resistance of bone to fracture. Bone strength depends upon bone structure. The more dense the trabecular pattern, the stronger is the bone. This compressive strength of the vertebral bodies decreases with age. See also: *Osteoporosis*.

Bone structural unit (BSU) Represents the end result of a remodeling cycle of mature bone. In cortical bone, it constitutes a Haversian system after a cortical remodeling unit has taken place. In cancellous bone, it is a wall or packet. See also: *Bone remodeling unit (BRU); Basic multicellular unit (BMU)*.

Bone substitute Nonviable biomaterial for reconstruction of bone, producing only a scaffold for formation of new bone. Supports the inherent potential for bone regeneration. It may be resorbable or remain in an unchanged version at the site of implantation. It also may assist in preservation of contour of an osseous reconstruction. See also: *Osteoconduction*.

Bone trap Device connected to the surgical suction to collect fine bone slurry within the surgical field during the drilling of bone or harvest of a bone block for alveolar ridge augmentation or maxillary sinus floor elevation. Collected bone can be added to the particulate graft.

Bone trephine Hollow, cylindrical cutting bur of various diameters used to harvest cylindrical bone blocks.

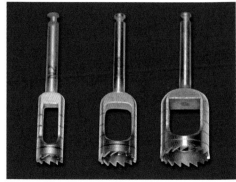

Bone trephine. (Courtesy of D. Buser)

Bony defect Alteration in the morphologic features of bone.

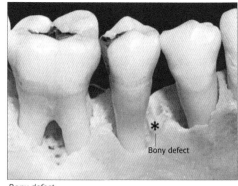

Bony defect.
(Reprinted from Rateitschack et al[38] with permission.)

Bovine-derived anorganic bone matrix Particular anorganic bovine bone substitute with a calcium-deficient carbonate hydroxyapatite having a crystal size of approximately 10 nm. All proteins are removed from the bovine xenograft via various chemical and physical processes. Its porous structure, like normal bone, is osteoconductive but resistant to resorption, although osteoclasts are identified in lacunae on the surfaces. The surface area is very large, and the modulus of elasticity is similar to that of normal bone.

Bovine hydroxyapatite material See: *Bovine-derived anorganic bone matrix*.

B

Bridge See: *Fixed prosthesis; Partial denture.*

BRU Abbreviation for *Bone remodeling unit.*

Brunski and Hurley model Set of equations that allows the user to predict the forces and moments acting on each implant in a group of implants that support a loaded prosthesis.[39]

Bruxism Involuntary grinding, clenching, or gnashing of teeth. This parafunctional activity may occur either diurnally or nocturnally and commonly results in excessive occlusal wear, periodontal trauma, pain, and neuromuscular problems. The etiology is not well understood but thought to be related to emotional stress and tension, occlusal irregularities, or central nervous system disorder.[7,40]

BSE Abbreviation for *Backscattered electron.* See: *Backscattered electron (BSE) imaging.*

BSU Abbreviation for *Bone structural unit.* See also: *Osteon.*

Buccal Related to the surface of the dental arch or posterior teeth adjacent to the cheek.[3]

Buccal mucosal incision Incision made in buccal nonkeratinized mucosa; not routinely used in implant surgery.

Bundle bone Bone of ectomesenchymal origin that lines the tooth alveolus and also forms the cribriform plate. It is characterized by perpendicular striations formed by the insertion of Sharpey fibers and blood vessels derived from the periodontal ligament. This tooth-related bone structure plays an important role during initial ridge alterations following extraction. Radiographically, it is called the *lamina dura.*[41]

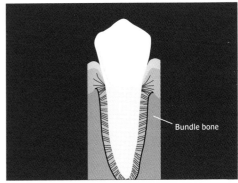

Bundle bone.
(Redrawn from Lindhe et al[42] with permission.)

Buser elevator Finely shaped instrument designed to gently elevate papillae and initiate flap elevation.

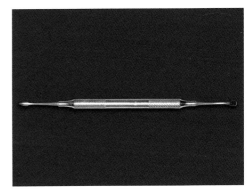

Buser elevator. (Courtesy of D. Buser)

Button implant See: *Mucosal insert.*

C

CAD/CAM   Acronym for computer-aided design/ computer-assisted manufacture.   See: *Computer-aided design/Computer-assisted manufacture (CAD/CAM).*

CAD/CAM abutment   Prosthetic implant component fabricated through the use of computer-aided design and/or computer-assisted manufacture (CAD/CAM).[1]

Calcified algae   Plants living in seawater, some in deep water, that are coral shaped with mineralized cell walls. *Corallina officinalis* (coral algae), used for the production of porous marine-derived coralline hydroxyapatite, is approximately 5 cm in height with built-in joint and belongs to the red algae group.   See also: *Porous marine-derived coralline hydroxyapatite.*

Calcified cartilage
See: *Endochondral ossification.*

Calcium carbonate
See: *Porous coralline hydroxyapatite.*

Calcium sulfate   Used in bone regeneration as an alloplastic graft, a graft binder, or a graft extender, and as a barrier. This biocompatible material ($CaSO_4$) resorbs following implantation. It has been shown that tissue will often migrate over calcium sulfate if primary closure cannot be obtained. Calcium sulfate has been proposed as a delivery vehicle for growth factors and antibiotics.[2-4]   See also: *Medical-grade calcium sulfate; Dental stone.*

Calculus   Hard concretion that forms on teeth or dental prostheses through calcification of bacterial plaque.[5]

Caldwell-Luc approach   Surgical approach using a window into the buccal bone wall of the maxillary sinus. The goal is sinus floor elevation to allow simultaneous or subsequent implant placement in sites with insufficient bone height.

Callus   Hard bony tissue that develops around the ends of a fractured bone during healing.[6]

Callus distraction   Basis for distraction osteogenesis in orthopedic surgery.   See also: *Distraction osteogenesis (DO).*

Calvarial bone   See: *Cranial bone.*

Calvarial bone harvest
See: *Cranial bone harvest.*

Calvarial graft   See: *Cranial bone harvest.*

Canaliculus   Minute canal extendig to the lacunae of bone   See: *Osteocyte.*

Cancellous bone   Composite of bone matrix and bone marrow. Osteoblasts, osteoprogenitor cells, and cytokines are transferred. Also used to describe a graft derived from cancellous bone, which is a spongy type of bone containing a trabecular structure with red bone marrow and most of the bone vasculature.   See also: *Trabecular bone.*

Cancer   See: *Neoplasm.*

C

Cancer reconstruction Tumor resection of the jaws often leads to discontinuity defects that need extensive bone reconstruction and restoration with implant-supported prostheses.

Canine guidance
See: *Canine-protected articulation.*

Canine-protected articulation Arrangement of teeth in which the vertical and horizontal overlap of the canines provide a guidance resulting in separation of the posterior teeth during eccentric movements of the mandible.[7]

Cantilever Extension on one end of a fixed prosthesis retained by single or multiple teeth or implants. Also used to describe a beam supported at one end only.[7,8]

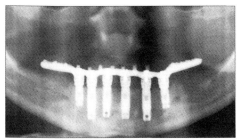

Cantilever.

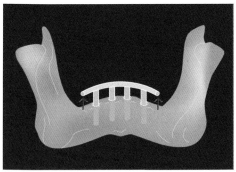

Cantilever.
(Reprinted from Watzek[9] with permission.)

Capillary Small terminal blood vessel connecting arterioles and venules.

Cartilage-derived morphogenetic protein 1 (CDMP1) Protein belonging to the transforming growth factor beta (TGF-β) superfamily involved in a variety of cellular functions. This molecule has been identified as one of the regulators of limb skeletogenesis and appendicular bone development.[10] See also: *Transforming growth factor beta (TGF-β).*

Case report Descriptive study of either a single patient or patient series that documents the patient's diagnosis, treatment, and management.[11,12]

Cast Three-dimensional image of an actual body part reproduced in a castable material.[2,13] See also: *Diagnostic cast; Master (definitive) cast; Preliminary cast.*

Castable abutment Prosthetic implant component made as a generic plastic pattern that can be designed or modified to specific dimensions. The pattern can be modified either by shaping via a rotary carbide bur or applying wax prior to alloy casting.

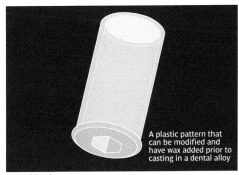

A plastic pattern that can be modified and have wax added prior to casting in a dental alloy

Castable abutment.

CAT Acronym for *computed axial tomography.* See: *Computed tomography (CT) scan.*

Cawood and Howell classification Classification of patterns of jaw bone atrophy serving to simplify description of the residual ridge. In the study published in 1988, it was found that the shape of the basilar process of the mandible and maxilla remains relatively stable, whereas changes in shape of the alveolar process are significant in both the vertical and horizontal axes and follow a predictable pattern.[14] See also: *Alveolar ridge, Classification of.*

CBA Abbreviation for *Cost-benefit analysis.*

CBFα1 Abbreviation for *Core-binding factor alpha 1.*

CDMP1 Abbreviation for *Cartilage-derived morphogenetic protein-1.*

CEA Abbreviation for *Cost-effectiveness analysis.*

Cell Microscopic mass of protoplasm enveloped by a semi-permeable membrane. Smallest structural unit of living matter able to function independently. See also: *Erythrocyte; B cell; Blood cell; Bone cell; Effector cell; Epithelial cell; Hematopoietic stem cell; Mesenchymal stem cell (MSC).*

Cell-occlusive membrane
See: *Barrier membrane.*

Cellular process All of the functions that cells perform to survive, including molecular transport, protein synthesis, DNA replication, reproduction, respiration, cellular metabolism, and signaling.

Cement Substance used to bind surfaces or objects together. Commonly stored as separate powder and liquid components that, when mixed together, become a luting agent upon hardening. To cement is to join surfaces by means of an appropriate medium.[2,3]

Permanent c. Binding or luting agent intended for long-term use, eg, zinc phosphate cement, which is composed of powder (zinc and magnesium oxides) and liquid (phosphoric acid, water, buffer agents). Other types include resin and glass–ionomer cements.

Temporary c. Binding or luting agent intended for short-term use, eg, zinc oxide (powder) eugenol (liquid) mixture.

Cement line Inactive bone surfaces are covered by a thin-density, stained 50-nm-thick line, consisting of a mineralized bone matrix in which the inorganic component is hydroxyapatite and the organics are proteoglycans and glycoproteins, with osteopontin as the major glycoprotein. The same line is apparent between implant surfaces and adjoining bone. Osteopontin functions as an adhesive and, in bone, binds collagen fibrils of new bone matrix to that of the old bone matrix.

Cementation Process involving the use of a binding substance to join surfaces to become a unit.[2]

Centric See: *Centric occlusion; Centric relation; Maxillomandibular relationship.*

Centric occlusion Positional relationship of occluding tooth surfaces when the mandible is in centric relation. The coincidence of centric occlusion and centric relation is desirable when creating an occlusion, but the maximal intercuspal relationship may not always exist.[3,15] See also: *Maxillomandibular relationship.*

Centric relation Clinically, the most retruded unstrained position of the mandibular condyles relative to the maxilla, from which lateral movements can be made at a given degree of jaw separation. Centric relation is a reference border position constant throughout life for each adult patient, provided the soft tissue structures in the temporomandibular joint are healthy. It is a reference relation from which a planned occlusal scheme can be coordinated.[16] See also: *Maxillomandibular relationship.*

Ceramic Crack-, heat-, and corrosion-resistant material fabricated from metal oxides of various sources. Also describes a field of research concerned with ceramic materials. See also: *Bioactive glass; Glass ceramic.*

Ceramic abutment Prosthetic implant component composed of a ceramic biomaterial that is considered an esthetic material as compared to unesthetic metal. The ceramic material used in fabrication of a prosthetic implant component varies as does the fabrication method of various manufacturers, which can include use of CAD/CAM technology.[17,18]

Ceramic crown One type of ceramic restoration. See also: *Ceramic restoration; Crown.*

Ceramic restoration Artificial substitute for tooth structure and anatomy fabricated entirely of ceramic material that covers and restores the remaining coronal portion of the tooth.

Cervix (pl: *cervices*) Constriction or narrowing of an object; sometimes referred to as the neck.[19] See also: *Implant neck.*

Chamfer Marginal tooth crown or implant abutment preparation creating a curve from the axial wall to the cavosurface.[3]

Chemotaxis Directed cell migration controlled by a biochemical concentration gradient.

Chemotherapy Use of chemical agents in the treatment or control of malignant disease. Patients undergoing chemotherapy are considered at high risk to develop postsurgical complications following implant placement.

Chewing See: *Mastication.*

Chewing cycle See: *Mandibular movement.*

Chin graft See: *Bone graft, Donor site for.*

Chisel Metal instrument with a tip that is beveled one side. Used in surgery to cut, cleave, or carve hard tissue. The shank can be straight or offset.[2]

Chi-square test Determines whether two attributes of the sample are independent or whether the presence of one is, in fact, associated with the presence of the other.[12]

Chlorhexidine Antibacterial compound ($C_{22}H_{30}Cl_{12}N_{10}$) that is a biguanide derivative used as a local antiseptic and disinfectant (eg, as in mouthwash) especially in the form of a hydrochloride, gluconate, or acetate.

Chondrocyte Mature cartilage-forming cell embedded in cartilage. Highly specialized connective tissue designed to withstand high compressive forces. Cartilage is nourished via diffusion. In endochondral ossification, the chondrocytes undergo apoptosis associated with vascularization, bone formation, and resorption of cartilage.

Chondroitin sulfate Plays a major role in maintaining the high osmotic tension essential to the elasticity of hyalin cartilage. Hyalin cartilage is composed of collagen type II that forms a meshwork, enclosing giant macromolecular aggregates of proteoglycans. Chondroitin sulfate is a main part of this ground substance.

Chronic abscess Abscess of comparatively slow development with minimal evidence of inflammation. Symptoms include intermittent discharge of purulent matter and long-standing collection of purulent exudate. May follow an acute abscess. Compare: *Residual abscess.*

Chronic infection Ongoing and often slowly progressing infection. Usually develops from an acute infection and can last for days to months to a lifetime.

Cicatrix   See: *Scar.*

Circulation, blood   General term for blood supply and flow through blood vessels, organs, and tissues.

Clamp, abutment   See: *Abutment clamp.*

Clamping force   Compressive force generated by bringing two distinct components together under pressure. It is created by external compressive forces or the tightening of a screw joint.

Cleft lip and/or palate   Most common craniofacial anomaly, occurring 1 in 600 to 700 live births, characterized by failure of fusion between embryologic processes during facial morphogenesis. Failure of fusion between the medial and lateral nasal and the maxillary processes results in a cleft of the lip and/or alveolar process, whereas failure of fusion between the lateral palatine processes results in a cleft of the palate. The cleft may be complete or incomplete, and it can occur unilaterally or bilaterally. Cleft lip may occur without clefting of the alveolar process or palate, and cleft palate can also occur as an isolated phenomenon.[20] (See figure.)

Clinical attachment level   Distance from the cementoenamel junction or implant collar to the tip of a periodontal probe during soft tissue diagnostic probing. Health of the attachment apparatus can affect the measurement.

Clinical implant performance scale   Quantitative scale to compare different implant systems in different indications, including the complications that occur and treatment procedures necessary in the aftercare period.[22]

Clip   See: *Attachment; Bar attachment system; Clip bar overdenture.*

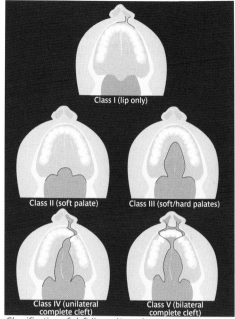

Classification of cleft lip and/or palate.
(Redrawn from Terkla and Laney[21] with permission.)

Clip bar overdenture   Overdenture prosthesis receiving partial retention from a bar clip. It is embedded in the impression surface of the restoration.   See also: *Implant overdenture.*

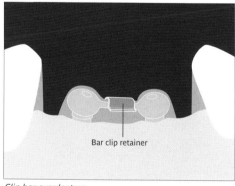

Clip bar overdenture.
(Redrawn from Brudvik[23] with permission.)

Closed curettage   Curettage performed via the gingival sulcus without flap reflection.[5]

Closed tray impression
See: *Indirect (closed tray) impression.*

Closure force Force generated by muscles of mastication. See also: *Biting force.*

Closure screw Surgical component inserted into the head of the implant or the occlusal surface of an implant. It is intended to obturate the access opening of the implant so as to prevent debris from flowing into or plugging the access. See also: *Cover screw.*

Clot See: *Blood clot.*

Coagulum See: *Blood clot.*

Coating Layer of material added to the surface of a structure; an additive surface.

Cohort study Study in which subjects who presently have a certain condition and/or receive a particular treatment are followed over time and compared with another group who are not affected by the condition under investigation.[24]

Col Valley-like depression of the interdental gingiva that connects facial and lingual papillae and conforms to the shape of the interproximal contact area.[5]

Cold-curing resin See: *Autopolymerizing resin.*

Collagen Insoluble fibrous protein of vertebrates that is the principal constituent of the fibrils of connective tissue and the organic substance of bones. Composed of tropocollagen molecules.

Collagen fleece Collagen-based biomaterial that improves hemostasis in surgery. It is essentially a collagen sponge coated with fibrinogen and thrombin to control bleeding in surgery.

Collagen membrane Resorbable barrier membrane made of heterogenic collagen, developed for guided tissue regeneration (GTR) or guided bone regeneration (GBR) techniques. The resorption time of collagen membranes can be controlled using methods of collagen cross-linking. See also: *Barrier membrane.*

Collagenase Matrix metalloproteinase enzymes that degrade collagen matrices derived from either the host or bacteria. See also: *Bacterial collagenase; Mammalian collagenase.*

Collar See: *Implant collar.*

Color matching Art and science of combining the attributes of color and color mixtures to include the properties of hue, value, saturation, opacity, translucency, and pigment loading.[25] See also: *Maxillofacial prosthetics.*

Comfort cap Element designed to fit over a component such as the transmucosal abutment. Intended to cover the component to protect the intraoral tissues from a detectible edge and/or prevent damage to the exposed surfaces of the component. See also: *Healing abutment.*

Commercially pure titanium (CPTi) Elemental titanium available commercially with residual contaminants (either accidental or intentional) that reduce the purity of the elemental titanium. More than a dozen grades of commercially pure titanium are available. Dental implants are most commonly fabricated from grades 1 through 4. See also: *Implant surface.*

Compact bone See: *Cortical bone.*

Compatible See: *Biocompatible.*

Compensating curve See: *Curve of Spee.*

Complete subperiosteal implant   See: *Subperiosteal implant.*

Complication   Unexpected deviation from the normal treatment outcome. It is generally classified as either technical or biological, eg, surgical complication, hemorrhage, damage to the inferior alveolar nerve, infection, delayed wound healing, or lack of osseointegration.   See also: *Esthetic complication.*

Component, implant
See: *Implant component.*

Composite graft   Graft composed of multiple graft types (eg, autogenous-synthetic graft or autogenous-xenograft), which may be mixed or layered within the defect.

Composite resin   Restorative resin usually formed by the reaction of an ether of bisphenyl-A with acrylic monomers initiated by a benzoyl peroxide-amine system. Additives include amorphous silica, glass beads or rods, quartz, and/or tricalcium phosphate.[2,3]

Compressive stress   Force directed toward the material being loaded.

Compromised bone   Bone impaired in quality and/or quantity as a result of cellular, vascular, or structural factors.[26]   See also: *Alveolar bone, Quality of; Alveolar bone, Quantity of.*

Compromised osteogenesis   Any interference with osteogenesis. Lack of primary stability during the placement of implants in the osteotomy site may lead to fibrous integration of the implant, instead of osseointegration, for example.

Computed axial tomography (CAT) scan
See: *Computed tomography (CT) scan.*

Computed tomography (CT) scan   Imaging method involving the narrow colimnation of a radiographic beam passing through human tis-

sues to be recorded by a variety of scintillation detectors. The collected information can then be digitally coordinated and displayed on a computer monitor or film. A CT scan must be performed to provide image data for a three-dimensional guidance system for implant placement.   See also: *Three-dimensional guidance system for implant placement.*

Computer-aided design/Computer-assisted manufacture (CAD/CAM)   Computer technology used to design and manufacture various components.

Computer-aided navigation   Computer system for intraoperative navigation, which provides the surgeon with current positions of the instruments and operation site on a three-dimensional reconstructed image of the patient that is displayed on a monitor in the operating room. The system aims to transfer preoperative planning on radiographs or computed tomography scans on the patient, in real-time, and independent of the position of the patient's head.

Computer-assisted manufacture surgical guidance   Computed tomography imaging augmented by implant placement planning to fabricate a surgical template for osteotomy localization during surgery.[27]

Configuration   Pattern or assembly method by which various elements and/or components are arranged. "The shape or outline of something, determined by the way its parts or elements are arranged."[28]

Congenital atresia   Congenital closure or absence of normal body opening or tubular structures.

Connecting bar   See: *Bar splint.*

Connection, abutment
See: *Abutment connection.*

Connective tissue Tissue of mesodermal origin consisting of various cells (eg, fibroblasts and macrophages) and interlacing protein fibers (eg, collagen) embedded in a chiefly carbohydrate ground substance that supports, ensheathes, and binds together other tissues. Includes loose and dense forms (eg, adipose tissue, tendons, ligaments, and aponeuroses) and specialized forms (eg, cartilage and bone). See also: *Fibrous connective tissue.*

Connective tissue attachment Union of connective tissue with the root surface. Original connective tissue attachment includes insertion of collagen fibers from the connective tissue into the radicular cementum.

Connective tissue graft Soft tissue augmentation procedure adopted from periodontal surgery using connective tissue harvested from a palatal donor site. See also: *Subepithelial connective tissue graft.*

Connector, intramobile
See: *Intramobile connector.*

Consensus General agreement or concord.

Consolidation period Final phase of distraction osteogenesis. Once the alveolar segment has been repositioned, the device is maintained in a static mode to act as a fixation device for a given amount of time.[29] See also: *Alveolar distraction osteogenesis.*

Construction See: *Prosthesis; Restoration.*

Contact osteogenesis Immediate primary apposition of woven bone on an implant surface as part of osseointegration. Compare: *Distance osteogenesis.*

Contraindication Any condition of the patient (ie, medical, psychological, or social) that makes a surgical procedure inadvisable.

Control See: *Examination.*

Conventional tomography Film tomography. Outdated in medicine, this imaging technique is of great interest in implant dentistry because it can be applied in private practice. The x-ray tube is rigidly fixed with a bar to the image receptor to move around a fixed axis. When a patient is properly positioned, objects located in this axis are projected on the same region in the image receptor and are clearly imaged. Objects located outside this axis are blurred. Thus, cross-sectional views can be obtained, for instance, of the maxilla and mandible to determine the width of the bone. Compare: *Computed tomography (CT) scan.*

Conversion prosthesis See: *Transitional prosthesis.*

Coolant Physiologic saline solution used to irrigate bone while during drilling procedures.

Coping In fixed prosthodontics, the metal substrate on which porcelain is applied in fabrication of a metal-ceramic restoration. Also used to describe the initial thin layer of wax on a die or a thin covering or crown.[30,31]

Coping design Specific coping shape or pattern, or the method by which it is made or planned. The coping is designed specifically for use within an implant system.

Coping screw Prosthetic component (ie, screw) incorporated as part of the anchorage by means of engaging threads so as to maintain the position of a coping (eg, impression coping). A one-piece element can also serve as the coping, which is threaded directly into the anchorage component. See also: *Prosthetic retaining screw.*

Coping, telescopic See: *Telescopic coping.*

Coral-derived hydroxyapatite Ca_2CO_3 skeleton of naturally occurring corals converted via a hydrothermic process to a non-biodegradable porous hydroxyapatite. See also: *Porous coralline hydroxyapatite; Porous marine-derived coralline hydroxyapatite.*

Corallina officinalis Calcifying marine algae. See also: *Calcified algae.*

Coralline See: *Porous coralline hydroxyapatite.*

Core-binding factor alpha 1 (CBFα1) An essential transcription factor for osteoblast differentiation and subsequent bone formation. Called also *runt-related transcription factor 2 (runx2)*. See also: *Bone morphogenetic protein (BMP).*

Corrective soft tissue surgery Plastic surgery procedure aimed at correcting either an inherited or acquired soft tissue defect. The surgery may include augmentation with a soft tissue graft (either connective tissue or free gingival graft) or correction of previous surgical scarring.

Correlation coefficient Measure of the linear association between two variables. It varies between +1 (perfect positive association) and −1 (perfect negative association). A value of 0 indicates that the two variables are not associated.[12]

Corrosion resistance Surface passivity rather than intrinsic unreactivity.

Corrugation Addition of parallel folds or grooves to a surface so as to increase the relative surface area or the stiffness of the material.

Cortical bone Consists of primary and secondary osteons with a periosteal and endosteal envelope. During growth, thickening and modeling of long bones takes place via pe-

riosteal deposition and endosteal resorption. In adulthood, a balance in shape and thickness is reached; in the elderly, the endosteal resorption may exceed the periosteal deposition, resulting in an increase in size of the marrow cavity and a decrease in cortical thickness. Primary osteons undergo continuous remodeling with formation of secondary osteons. Growth factors are released as part of the resorptive process of autografts. See also: *Bone remodeling.*

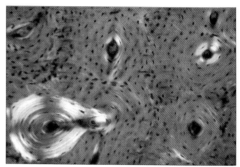

Cortical bone (polarized light; magnification x125). (Reprinted from Buser et al[32] with permission.)

Cortical bone graft See: *Bone graft.*

Corticocancellous bone Graft derived from donor sites with both cortical and cancellous components, such as the symphysis or iliac crest. Autogenous origin of this type of bone graft is ideal because of the mechanical stability, the inherent supply of bone morphogenetic proteins (BMPs) in cortical bone, and the osteogenic potential of cancellous bone.

Corticocancellous bone graft See: *Bone graft.*

Corticosteroid See: *Glucocorticoid.*

Corticotomy Partial osteotomy involving only the cortical plate; used in distraction osteogenesis to separate the transporting segment.

Cosmetic periodontal surgery   Surgical periodontal procedures to improve gingival esthetics and achieve an ideal soft tissue-teeth relationship. It includes treatment of gingival recession, gingivectomy and gingivoplasty.   See also: *Gingival recession; Gingivectomy; Gingivoplasty*.

Cost analysis   Investigation and examination of factors related to the value.

Cost-benefit analysis (CBA)   Study designed to assess all outcomes based on monetary costs and benefits. All study results are conveyed in dollars or euros. An economic conversion is used to express a monetary amount to intangible results.[12]

Cost-effectiveness analysis (CEA)   Study comparing two or more therapies on the bases of monetary costs and clinical effectiveness. Results are usually reported in units of dollars or euros per clinical outcome. The outcome of therapies to be compared with CEA must be expressed in the same units.[12]

Countersinking   Bone preparation of the crestal area using special countersinking drills to allow an apical implant placement resulting in a subcrestal position of the implant shoulder or platform.

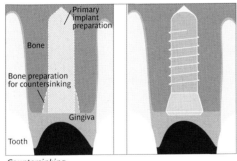

Countersinking.

Cover screw   Screw with head design to fit over the implant and seal the occlusal surface of the implant prior to wound closure in a two-stage surgical implant procedure.   See also: *Closure screw.*

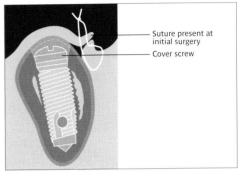

Cover screw.

CPTi   Abbreviation for *Commercially pure titanium.*

Cranial bone   Bone taken from any of the bones surrounding the brain, comprising the paired bones (ie, parietal and temporal) and the unpaired bones (ie, occipital, frontal, sphenoid, and ethmoid). Called also *calvarial bone.*

Cranial bone harvest   Any of the bones surrounding the brain; the paired parietal and temporal bones and the unpaired occipital, frontal sphenoid, and ethmoid bones.[33]

Craniofacial implant
See: *Percutaneous implant.*

Craniofacial implant prosthesis   See: *Craniofacial prosthesis.*

Craniofacial prosthesis   Extraoral restoration replacing a portion of the cranium or face and retained by skin-penetrating implants or adhesives.   See also: *Maxillofacial prosthetics.*

Crater   Saucer-shaped defect of soft tissue or bone often seen interdentally.[5]   See also: *Bony defect.*

Craterization See: *Paracervical saucerization.*

Creep Property of a material, usually metal, to deform or elongate under pressure that is either cyclic or constant.

Creeping substitution See: *Bone remodeling.*

Crest Peak or top of an edentulous alveolar ridge.

Crestal bone loss See: *Atrophic alveolar bone.*

Crestal incision Incision placed at the crest or on top of the alveolar ridge of an edentulous space.

Crevicular epithelium Epithelial lining of the gingival crevice, sulcus, or periodontal pocket; generally a stratified squamous epithelium. Called also *sulcular epithelium.*

Crevicular fluid See: *Gingival crevicular fluid (GCF).*

Crevicular physiologic dimension
See: *Biologic width.*

Critical-sized defect Smallest osseous defect that will never heal completely with osseous tissue components. The size varies according to species and anatomic location of the primary defect.

Cross-arch stabilization Counteraction to prosthesis unseating forces provided by natural teeth or implants on the opposite side of the arch. This resistance may be provided by splinted or fixed prosthetic units or components of a removable partial prosthesis.[3,34] See also: *Splinting.*

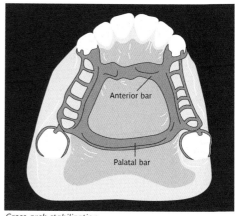

Cross-arch stabilization.
(Redrawn from McGivney and Castleberry[35] with permission.)

Cross-bite occlusion Occluding tooth contact in which the natural or artificial mandibular teeth overlap the maxillary teeth. Called also *reverse articulation.*[2,3]

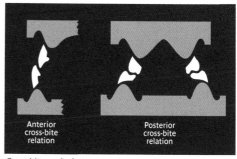

Cross-bite occlusion.
(Redrawn from Boucher[36] with permission.)

Cross-sectional study Study done at one time, not over the course of time. A cross-sectional study of a disease (eg, aggressive periodontitis) completed at a single point in time reveals the prevalence and distribution of the disease within a defined population. Called also *synchronic study.*[37]

Crown Highest part of an object, such as with the normally exposed part of a natural tooth covered by enamel, or an artificial restoration replacing part or all of the coronal portion of a tooth or implant abutment for esthetic and functional purposes.[2,3] See also: *Acrylic restoration; Ceramic restoration.*

Crown-implant ratio Relation between the length of the restoration (ie, crown) and the length of the implant embedded in bone. The crown is measured from the most coronal bone contact to the most coronal surface of the restoration and the implant is measured from the implant apex to the most coronal bone contact.[3,34]

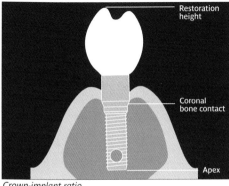

Crown-implant ratio.
(Redrawn from Brånemark et al[38] with permission.)

CT Abbreviation for *computed tomography*. See: *Computed tomography (CT) scan.*

C-telopeptide pyridinoline cross-links of type I collagen Pyridinoline cross-links represent a class of mature collagen degradative molecules that include pyridinoline, deoxypyridinoline, N-telopeptides, and C-telopeptides. Following procollagen synthesis and release into the maturing extracellular matrix, pyridinoline cross-links are formed in type I collagen by the enzyme lysyl oxidase on lysine and hydroxylysine residues in the carboxy- and amino-terminal telopeptide regions, increasing the mechanical stability of the structure. Subsequent to osteoclastic bone resorption and collagen matrix degradation, cross-linked telopeptides of type I collagen are released into the circulation. Since cross-linked telopeptides result from posttranslational modification of collagen molecules, they cannot be reused during collagen synthesis and are therefore precise indicators of bone resorption. C-terminal telopeptides of type I collagen (ICTP) have been identified as biomarkers of bone resorption and bone turnover in a variety of osseous metabolic diseases including osteoporosis, rheumatoid arthritis, periodontal disease, and peri-implant disease.

Cumulative success rate Estimate of the proportion of successful implants based on a predefined set of criteria, from baseline to time of interest. See also: *Life table analysis.*

Cumulative survival rate Estimate of the proportion of successful implants that have not led to tooth or implant loss, from baseline to time of interest. See also: *Life table analysis.*

Cuneiform Wedge-shaped.

Curet or curette Instrument used to debride tissue. In periodontics, a curet is used for scaling and planing of tooth roots or implant surfaces and for debridement (also called *curettage*) of periodontal pockets and bone.

Curettage Scraping or cleaning of the walls of a cavity or surface by means of a curet.[5] See also: *Bone curettage; Closed curettage; Gingival curettage; Open curettage.*

Curve of Spee Curved line produced by connecting the tip of the natural mandibular canine with the buccal cusps of the premolars and molars and extended to the anterior border of the mandibular ramus. This anatomic observation was first made by F. G. Spee in the 19th century. In the absence of natural teeth, this curve is developed to compensate for condylar path influence on occlusal contacts in the creation of a balanced occlusion; hence the term *compensating curve.*[2,3]

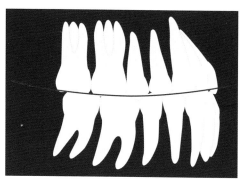

Curve of Spee (compensating curve).
(Redrawn from Daskalogiannakis[20] with permission.)

Cusp　Peaked extension of the occlusal surface of a molar or premolar. Cusp incline is determined by the mesiodistal or buccolingual slope from the peak to the deepest part of the central fossa of the tooth.[3]

Cusp inclination　Relative cusp height of artificial teeth; affects the loading pattern of a supporting dental implant.

Custom abutment
See: *Castable abutment; UCLA abutment.*

Cutis　See: *Skin.*

Cutting cone　See: *Bone remodeling unit (BRU); Basic multicellular unit (BMU).*

Cutting torque　Turning or twisting force produced by a rotary device (ie, dental handpiece) to cut through a material such as bone.

Cylinder-to-transmucosal element　See: *Gold cylinder attachment.*

Cylinder wrench　Instrument used clinically and can be modified for use in dental laboratory implant procedures. It is designed by the manufacturer to fit specific prosthetic components and used to adjust the component.

Cylindrical implant　Implant of variable design and configuration, depending on the implant system. One such design, determined either in cross-section or three-dimension, follows the shape of a cylinder for an endosteal implant.

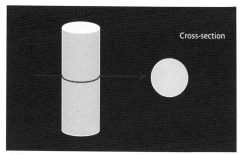

Cylindrical implant (cross section view of a cylinder).

Cytokine　Growth factor that stimulates growth and differentiation via cellular receptors. Examples are platelet-derived growth factor (PDGF), insulin growth factors (IGS), transforming growth factor beta 1 (TGF-β1), bone morphogenetic proteins (BMPs), and epidermal growth factor (EGF).

Cytotoxic　Cell toxicity; the capacity to kill cells.

Cytotoxin　Agent that has toxic effects on cells or inhibits or prevents cell function.

D

DBM   Abbreviation for *Demineralized bone matrix*.

Debridement   Removal of inflamed, devitalized, or contaminated tissue or foreign material from or adjacent to a lesion.

Deciduous dentition   See: *Dentition, primary*.

Decortication   Intraoperative preparation of the recipient bone bed by making numerous small perforations into the cortex to induce bleeding from the marrow cavity. This technique is routinely used in combination with onlay block grafts or guided bone regeneration (GBR) procedures.   See also: *Bone preparation*.

Defect   Genetic or acquired deficiency of an anatomic structure (ie, bone or soft tissue) required for normal function or esthetics.   See also: *Critical-sized defect*.

Definitive cast   See: *Master impression*.

Definitive prosthesis   Orodental or maxillofacial restoration designed and fabricated for long-term use. This term is preferable to *final prosthesis*, since no artificial replacement can be considered permanent.[1]

Dehiscence   Buccal or lingual bone defect in the crestal area extending apically at an implant.   See also: *Fenestration; Wound dehiscence*.

Delayed implant placement   See: *Late implant placement*.

Delayed loading   Placing an implant into function or a load-bearing situation following an extended period of healing after the initial placement.

Demineralized bone matrix (DBM)   Bone matrix, usually allogeneic in origin, that may induce bone formation via release of growth factors and bone morphogenetic proteins (BMPs) from the matrix, occasionally after osteoclastic breakdown. Osteoinductive potential may vary, dependent on method of preparation and degree of demineralization.

Demineralized freeze-dried bone allograft (DFDBA)   By demineralization, the mineral phase of freeze-dried bone allografts is partly or completely removed so that the collagen and non-collagenous matrix is exposed, thereby making growth factors available.

Dental cast   See: *Cast*.

Dental plaster
  See: *Calcium sulfate; Dental stone*.

Dental stone   Denser alpha-hemihydrate form of calcium sulfate, stronger than the beta form. It is commonly used for dental casts involved in the fabrication of denture prostheses. An even denser, stronger die stone is used to create a positive likeness of a prepared tooth for the fabrication of crown restorations.[1]   See also: *Calcium sulfate*.

Dentition   Collective teeth in the dental arches.[2,3]

  Artificial d.   Imitation replacement for natural teeth.

Natural d. Normal living teeth that erupt into the oral cavity.

Permanent d. Natural teeth that succeed the primary teeth as the primary teeth are shed. Called also *succedaneous dentition*.

Primary d. Earliest natural teeth that erupt into the dental arches of the oral cavity normally during childhood. Called also *deciduous dentition*.

Dentoalveolar distraction See: *Alveolar distraction osteogenesis*.

Dentofacial orthopedics See: *Orthodontics*.

Denture Artificial replacement for natural teeth and related structures. A *conventional* or *traditional denture* is a generic phrase for the long-standing concept of a dental prosthesis, most commonly a removable prosthesis.[2] See also: *Prosthesis*.

Denture prosthesis A generic term for the long-standing concept of artificial replacement of natural teeth and related structures, most commonly a removable device. The term is also used to denote its distinctness from an implant-supported or a craniofacial prosthesis.[1,2]

De-osseointegration State in which prior osseointegration is subsequently lost.

Depassivation Removal or loss of an oxide layer from the surface of a metal.

Deproteinized bovine bone material See: *Bovine-derived anorganic bone matrix*.

Depth gauge Gauge for measuring the depth of grooves or holes or other concavities. In implant dentistry, used to measure the depth of the osteotomy during implant site preparation.

Dermal graft Skin graft made with a thin split-thickness graft of dermis.[4] See also: *Acellular dermal allograft*.

Developmental anomaly Aberration in the normal sequence of events associated with growth and development. This process could result over time in distortion of the face and jaws, abnormality of tooth formation or position, and irregularity of function.[2,5]

Device Apparatus, instrumentation, or machine designed to carry out a specific purpose.

DFDBA Abbreviation for *Demineralized freeze-dried bone allograft*.

Diabetes mellitus (DM) Encompasses a heterogeneous group of disorders with the common characteristic of altered glucose tolerance or impaired lipid and carbohydrate metabolism. DM develops from either a deficiency in insulin production or an impaired utilization of insulin. Based on these two conditions, DM can be divided into Type 1 (formerly *insulin-dependent diabetes mellitus*) and Type 2 (formerly *non-insulin-dependent diabetes*).[6]

Diabetes mellitus – related surgical risk factors Surgical risk factors for a diabetic patient include intraoperative hypo- or hyperglycemia and delayed postoperative wound healing. Such patients may also be more susceptible to infection.[6,7]

Diagnostic Pertaining to any measure used for the purpose of diagnosis.

Diagnostic cast Reproduction of actual teeth and associated oral structures used for analysis and treatment planning.[1,2]

Diagnostic imaging Visual representation of a body part made for diagnostic and/or treatment planning purposes. Such procedures include radiography, computed tomography (CT), magnetic resonance imaging (MRI), ultrasound, and digital volume tomography.

Diagnostic wax-up Arrangement of artificial teeth or waxed occlusal and incisal surfaces created in the laboratory for evaluation of projected prosthetic restorations. The accepted arrangement can be used for treatment planning, surgical or radiographic template fabrication, and prosthesis design.[8]

Diaphysis Shaft of long bones, consisting of compact bone and bone marrow cavity.

Digital prosthesis Artificial replacement for human fingers, including the thumb. See also: *Maxillofacial prosthetics.*

Direct (open tray) impression Impression technique by which an occlusal opening is created in a fabricated custom tray that permits impression coping removal with the impression material as a single unit.[8]

Direction indicator Device that fits into the osteotomy or implant at the time of surgical placement. When two indicators are placed in adjacent osteotomies or implants, the relative parallelism can be evaluated and additional corrective procedures can be accomplished at the surgical stage.

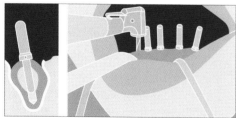

Direction indicator.

Disarticulation See: *Disocclusion.*

Disclosant Dye (tablet or solution) used to stain dental biofilm. It is primarily used as an aid in oral hygiene instruction for dental plaque identification and enables the patient to determine the effectiveness of his or her oral care routine.

Disclusion See: *Disocclusion.*

Disk implant Interpositional implant used for placement in joints such as the temporomandibular joint following a meniscectomy. Various materials have been used to fabricate interpositional implants including polytetrafluoroethylene (PTFE), an alloplastic material. Also, a disk made of commercially pure titanium that is designed with concave-shaped ovoid perforations and "inserted from the lateral aspect of the host bone and provides multicortical support." Additional anchorage is achieved using an axial direction by threading a screw-type implant through the central opening of the multiple disks.[9]

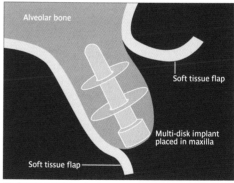

Endosseous disk implant.

Disocclusion Separation of the mandible from the maxilla precipitated by tooth-guided contacts during mandibular excursive movements. Called also *disclusion* or *disarticulation.*[10]

Distal extension   Edentulous space posterior to the most distal tooth or implant abutment.

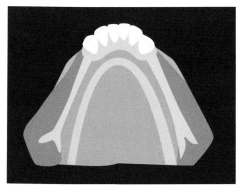

Distal extension (mandibular).

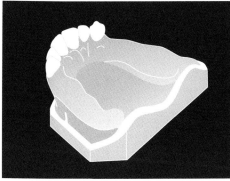

Distal extension (maxillary).

Distal extension prosthesis   As seen in the median sagittal plane, a prosthesis addition posterior to the most distal tooth or implant abutment. The extension can be uni- or bilateral and in the form of an artificial tooth or teeth, a cantilever for a fixed prosthesis, or a denture base segment for a removable partial denture.[1]   See also: *Partial denture.*

Distance osteogenesis   Immediate primary apposition of woven bone on the surface of the osseous implant bed as part of the osseointegration process.   Compare: *Contact osteogenesis*.

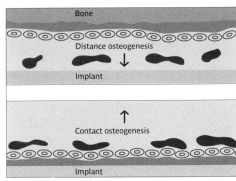

Distance osteogenesis.
(Redrawn from Schenk et al[11] with permission.)

Distraction, bidirectional crest   See: *Bidirectional crest distraction.*

Distraction device   See: *Distractor.*

Distraction implant   Distraction device that incorporates an implant into its design. The implant may then be used for prosthetic reconstruction following distraction.

Distraction osteogenesis (DO)   Surgical process for reconstruction of skeletal deformities that involves gradual, controlled displacement of surgically created fractures to simultaneously expand soft tissue and bone volume. In this approach to maxillary and mandibular augmentation, a favorable mechanical strain is applied to the healing callus in the osteotomy gap, usually a week after osteotomy. By gradual traction (1 mm per day) the height may be increased by 10 mm or more. Gavriel Ilizarov, a Russian orthopedic surgeon, is credited with developing the technique for orthopedic limb deformities in the 1960s. These concepts have been modified for use in maxillofacial surgery.[12]   See also: *Alveolar distraction osteogenesis.*

Distraction rate   Distance of distraction per day. Ideal rate depends on the ability of the soft tissue to respond with expansion and regeneration. Periodontal status of adjacent teeth may also limit the transport rate. In general, a rate of 0.4 mm per day is sufficient to allow the soft tissue to respond while avoiding premature consolidation (ie, fusion) across the vertical osteotomy components prior to completion of the transport process. If the distraction rate is too slow, the risk for premature consolidation is increased.[12]   See also: *Distraction osteogenesis (DO)*.

Distraction regenerate   Newly regenerated tissue between the transported section and the surgically cut base achieved following distraction osteogenesis (DO).   See also: *Alveolar distraction osteogenesis.*

Distraction rhythm   Number of increments of distraction given over a day.   See also: *Distraction rate.*

Distraction vector   Three-dimensional direction in which the transported section is guided in distraction osteogenesis (DO).

Distraction zone   Zone between the transported segment and its surgically cut base.

Distractor   Device used for distraction osteogenesis (DO).   See also: *Alveolar distraction osteogenesis; Distraction osteogenesis (DO); Intraoral distractor.*

   Endosseous d.   See: *Endosseous distractor.*

   Extraosseous d.   See: *Extraosseous distractor.*

Distribution force   Pattern in which applied forces are distributed throughout a structure; ie, pattern of load distribution throughout an implant-supported fixed cantilever prosthesis.

Disuse   In bone, the relationship between the bone's strength and its usual imposed loads. Disuse-mode remodeling results in local removal of bone.   See also: *Disuse atrophy*.

Disuse atrophy   Wasting away or degeneration in any bone from lack of normal functional stimulus; ie, bone loss in paraplegia or alveolar bone loss after tooth extraction.

DM   Abbreviation for *Diabetes mellitus*.

DO   Abbreviation for *Distraction osteogenesis*.

Dolder bar   Prefabricated U-shaped bar used to connect teeth, tooth roots, or implant abutments to provide support and retention. The retentive feature of this design is a single sleeve incorporated in the impression surface of the prosthesis. The bar has two basic shapes: an egg-shaped bar allows movement, whereas a modified bar unit is rigid.[13,14]

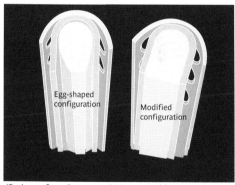

(Redrawn from Brewer and Morrow[14] with permission.)

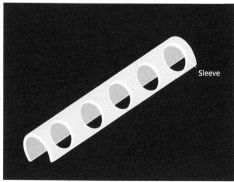

Dolder bar configurations and sleeve.

D

Donor site   See: *Bone graft, Donor site for.*

Doxycycline   Semisynthetic broad-spectrum antibacterial of the tetracycline group, administered orally. This antibiotic is often used to treat periodontal and peri-implant disease. Low-dose formulations also possess inhibitory effects on matrix metalloproteinase (MMP) enzymes responsible for destroying connective tissues and bone.

Dressing   Application of a gauze or bandage to cover and protect a sore, ulcer, or wound.   See also: *Periodontal dressing.*

Drill extender   Intermediate handpiece or wrench component used to lengthen the shaft of an instrument connected to a rotary drill or implant mount.[8]

Drill guide   A template, sleeve, other device, or system used to direct/control a rotary cutting instrument when preparing an implant osteotomy site.   See also: *Computed tomography (CT) scan; Three-dimensional guidance system for implant placement.*

Drilling sequence   Sequence of a series of burs and drills to methodically prepare an implant site.

Dual-energy x-ray absorptiometry (DEXA)   Means of measuring bone mineral density (BMD). It is the most widely used and most thoroughly studied bone density measurement technology. Bone density can be measured in every part of the body, preferably in rib and vertebra, and has been measured as well in the jaw area. The patient's bone is exposed to two x-ray beams of different energy levels. The absorption of each beam by bone is correlated with the quantity of calcium crystals per volume. The value of absorption calculates the bone density in mg/cm^2. The drawback of the method is that soft tissue absorption is subtracted out and the value of cortical bone and bone marrow has to be determined by integral calculus. The effective radiation dose to the patient per examination has been calculated as 0.01 mSv.

Dynamic loading   Situation in which the loading of an implant is continually changing as would happen during occlusal function. Both the magnitude and direction of applied force are in constant flux.

Dysesthesia   Unpleasant abnormal sensation, which can be spontaneous or evoked.

E

Ear prosthesis Fixed/removable artificial replacement for all or part of a human ear. Called also *auricular prosthesis*.

Early implant loss Loss of an implant that occurs prior to implant osseointegration.

Early implant placement Early implant placement takes place 4 to 8 weeks following tooth extraction, providing sufficient time for soft tissue healing. This approach is often used by clinicians in esthetic sites, where implant placement often requires a simultaneous guided bone regeneration (GBR) procedure and primary soft tissue closure is critical. It helps to reduce the risk of post-restorative soft tissue complications. [1]

Early loading Placing of an implant into function or a load-bearing situation following a reduced period of healing after the initial placement. It is generally considered to be loading more than 48 hours but less than 3 months after implant placement.[2]

Eccentric See: *Maxillomandibular relationship, Eccentric.*

ECM Abbreviation for *Extracellular matrix.*

Edentulism Oral condition of being without teeth, completely (ie, complete edentulism) or in segments of a dental arch (ie, partial edentulism).

Edentulous Without teeth.

Edentulous space Space interval between teeth that was previously occupied by a tooth or teeth.

EDM Abbreviation for *Electric discharge method.*

Effector cell Cell that becomes active in response to stimulation. In immunology, a differentiated lymphocyte capable of mounting a specific immune response, eg, antibody production; lymphokine production; or helper, suppressor, or killer function. Called also *effector lymphocyte.*

Effector lymphocyte See: *Effector cell.*

EGF Abbreviation for *Epidermal growth factor.*

Elastic modulus Measure of elasticity; relative stiffness of a material within the range of elastic deformation (below the point of plastic deformation). Called also *modulus of elasticity* or *Young modulus.*

Elastic modulus = Stress/Strain or $E = \sigma/\varepsilon$

Electric discharge method (EDM) Fabrication of components through use of electrically induced contact corrosion. Called also *spark erosion.*

Element Separate, identifiable part or a distinct group within a larger group; ie, any portion of an implant prosthesis. It can be identified by position or function as transmucosal, retentive, attachment, or dental.[3,4]

Elevator   Surgical instrument. A luxating elevator is used to luxate teeth during extraction. A periosteal elevator is used to elevate a full-thickness or mucoperiosteal flap.

Buser e.   See: *Buser elevator*.

EMD   Abbreviation for *Enamel matrix derivative*.

Emergence angle   Angle formed by the surface of the transmucosal element to the long axis of the implant.[5]   See also: *Emergence profile*. (See figure.)

Emergence profile   Facial or buccal axial contour of a tooth or crown, extending from the base of the epithelial sulcus past the soft tissue margin to the height of contour. Control of this surface is important in achieving acceptable esthetics and maintaining soft tissue health.[6,7]   See also: *Emergence angle*.

Enamel matrix derivative (EMD)   Extract of embryonic enamel matrix derived from six-month-old piglets. It is composed of several proteins, 90% of which are amelogenins, a family of hydrophobic proteins. EMD has been used as a periodontal regenerative treatment.

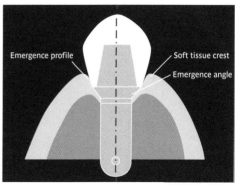

Emergence angle and emergence profile. (Redrawn from Yanase and Preston[7] with permission.)

Endochondral ossification   Formation of long bones on the basis of a cartilaginous model. Longitudinal growth takes place both in growth plates and in the articular cartilage. At the growth plates, chondral ossification takes place. Cartilage cells calcify, serving as a basis for bone formation, and bone is deposited; cartilage is then replaced by bone.

Endocrine   Transfer of chemical compounds such as hormones and growth factors from secreting glands via blood to cells.

Endodontic pin   See: *Endodontic stabilizer*.

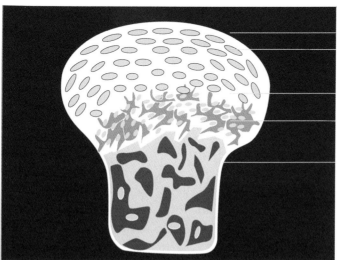

Fibrous layer (type I collagen)
Zone of proliferation of prechondrocytes

Zone of biosynthesis of type II collagen and large prostaglandins

Zone of hypertrophic chondrocytes and cartilage mineralization

Zone of bone formation

Endochondral ossification. (Redrawn from Garant[8] with permission.)

Endodontic stabilizer   Tapered post made of a biocompatible alloy that is cemented into a natural tooth, extending beyond the apex into the surrounding bone, on the assumption that it would stabilize the tooth.[9] Called also *endodontic pin*.

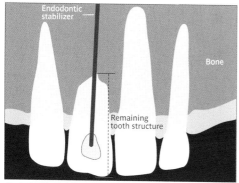

Endodontic stabilizer.

Endosseous distractor   Distraction device designed to be placed within bone, between the bone base and transport segment.   See also: *Distraction osteogenesis (DO)*.

Endosseous implant   Relative bony anatomic position of an implant placed into an osteotomy site. "A device placed into the alveolar and/or basal bone of the mandible or maxilla and transsecting only one cortical plate." Classification term *endosseous* is interchangeable with the term *endosteal*.[10]

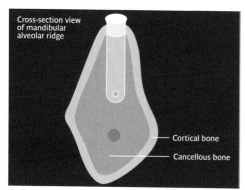

Endosseous implant.

Endosseous provisional implant   See: *Provisional implant*.

Endosseous ramus implant   Single- or multiple-piece implant in which the endosseous elements are placed in the symphysis area and into the anterior portion of bilateral mandibular rami. The transmucosal element extends from the endosseous portion that supports a mesostructure. The mesostructure can consist of a bar that follows the general outline of the residual mandibular bone. It is U-shaped as viewed from the occlusal.[11-13]

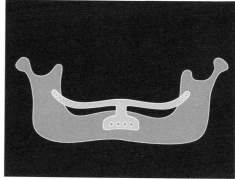

Endosseous ramus implant.

Endosteal   Synonym for *endosseous*.   See also: *Intraosseous*.

Endosteum   Thin, vascular membrane that lines the inner aspect of cortical bone surrounding the medullary cavity of bone. This delicate connective tissue is comprised of vessels, lining cells, and osteoprogenitor cells and has a marked osteogenic potential.

Endothelial progenitor cell   Adherent cell obtained from peripheral blood-derived or bone marrow – derived mononuclear cells demonstrating low-density lipoprotein (LDL) uptake and isolectin-binding capacity. These cells may be used as a potential therapy for a variety of vascular diseases. The number of circulating endothelial progenitor cells is reduced in patients with cardiovascular disease and may be a surrogate marker for this disease risk.[14]

E

Endothelium (pl: *endothelia*) Epithelium of mesoblastic origin composed of a single layer of thin, flattened cells that line the cavities of the heart, the lumina of blood and lymph vessels, and the serous cavities of the body.

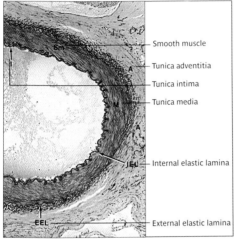

Smooth muscle
Tunica adventitia
Tunica intima
Tunica media
Internal elastic lamina
External elastic lamina

Endothelium. (Photomicrograph; magnification x122; elastic stain.)
(Reprinted from Berman[15] with permission.)

Endotoxin Potentially toxic, natural compounds found inside pathogens such as bacteria. Unlike an exotoxin, it is not secreted in soluble form by live bacteria but is a structural component in the bacteria that is released mainly when bacteria are lysed. Endotoxin is associated with the outer membranes of certain gram-negative bacteria, and its main active ingredient is the lipopolysaccharide (LPS) or lipo-oligo-saccharide (LOS) complex. It can

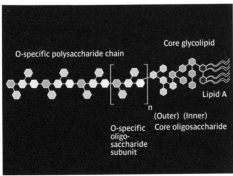

O-specific polysaccharide chain
Core glycolipid
Lipid A
n
(Outer) (Inner)
O-specific oligo-saccharide subunit
Core oligosaccharide

Endotoxin.

be cytotoxic or pyogenic, has been shown to induce and/or amplify inflammation, and has been implicated in the etiologies of periodontitis. For most purposes, the terms endotoxin and lipopolysaccharide (LPS) are used interchangeably. See also: *Lipopolysaccharide (LPS).*

Envelope flap Flap that is elevated without vertical releasing incisions, thus creating an envelope or pouch; most often used in combination with connective tissue grafts.

Epidermal cell Any of the cells making up the epidermis, the outer layer of the skin covering the exterior body surface. Epidermis comprises, from within, five epithelial layers: the basal layer (stratum basale), the spinous layer (stratum spinosum), the granular layer (stratum granulosum), the clear layer (stratum lucidum), and the cornified layer (stratum corneum).

Epidermal growth factor Mitogenic polypeptide that promotes growth and differentiation, is essential in embryogenesis, and is important in wound healing. [16]

Epiphysis End of a bone shaft, consisting of trabecular bone covered by a thin cortex.

Epithelial apical migration Migration of gingival sulcular and junctional epithelia in the apical direction as a result of periodontitis progression. During the healing process after periodontal therapy, the epithelial cells migrate apically attaching to the root or oral implant surface and preventing connective tissue cell attachment.

Epithelial attachment
See: *Junctional epithelium.*

Epithelial cell Cell that lines hollow organs and glands and that makes up the outer surface of the body. Arranged in single or multiple layers, depending on the type, they help protect or enclose organs. Some produce mucus or other secretions, and others have tiny hairs called cilia, which help remove foreign substances, for example, from the respiratory tract.

Epithelial implant   See: *Mucosal insert.*

Epithelialization   Healing by growth of epithelium over connective tissue.

Epithelialized palatal graft   See: *Free gingival graft.*

Epithelium   (pl: *epithelia*)   Covering of internal and external surfaces of the body, including the lining membrane of vessels and other small cavities. It consists of cells joined by small amounts of cementing substances and is classified on the basis of the number of layers deep and the shape of the superficial cells.   See also: *Crevicular epithelium; Junctional epithelium.*

Epithesis (prosthesis)   Craniofacial artificial replacement supported and retained by percutaneous (epi) implants.[17]   See also: *Maxillofacial prosthetics.*

Eposteal implant   Implant that rests on and is directly supported by bone.[6]   Compare: *Subperiosteal implant.*

Epoxy resin   Resin molecule characterized by reactive epoxy or ethoxyline groups serving as terminal polymerization points. It is used in dentistry as denture base material and is versatile in its capacity to adhere to wood, glass, and metal.

e-PTFE   Abbreviation for *Expanded polytetrafluoroethylene.*

Epulis   (pl: *epulides*)   Nonspecific term applied to tumors and tumor-like masses of the gingiva; peripheral ossifying fibroma.

Er:YAG laser   Er:YAG is an acronym for *erbium-doped yttrium aluminum garnet*, a compound that is used as the lasing medium for certain solid-state lasers. Er:YAG lasers typically emit light with a wavelength of 2,940 nm, which is in the infrared range. The frequency of Er:YAG lasers is at the resonant frequency of water, which causes it to be quickly absorbed; this limits its use in surgery.

Erythrocyte   Mature red blood cell. The function of this nonnucleated, biconcave disk containing hemoglobin is to transport oxygen.

Esthetic complication   Complication caused by the malposition of an implant in either the mesiodistal, coronal-apical, or orofacial direction, or by the lack of peri-implant bone or soft tissues. Such complications can be a major concern for clinicians, since removal of the implant may be required.[18]

Esthetic zone   Teeth or restorations and their associated supporting structures that are visible when exposed by patient smile.[6,19]

Esthetics   Beauty or physical appearance provided by the form and composition of the teeth, mouth, and face.[20]   See also: *Esthetic zone.*

Etched surface   See: *Acid-etched implant.*

Etching   Act of creating an etched surface through the application of corrosive chemicals, usually acids. It is considered beneficial for the promotion of osseointegration.   See also: *Acid etching.*

Examination   Process of assessing a body part or parts to ascertain the state of health or disease; may include visualization, digital palpation, percussion, auscultation, radiographic analysis, ultrasound, and/or other laboratory and functional measurement techniques. The examination can be preoperative for diagnostic purposes or postoperative for treatment follow-up. Called also *control.*[20]

Exclusion criterion   (pl: *exclusion criteria*)   Condition that precludes entrance of candidates into an investigation, even if they meet the inclusion criteria.   Compare: *Inclusion criterion.*

Exenteration   Removal of an organ. For maxillofacial prosthetics, removal of the eye and surrounding contents from the orbit, called *orbital exenteration*; usually implies the fabrication of an orbital prosthesis.[21]

Exfoliation   Physiologic shedding or loss of a primary tooth prior to the eruption of its permanent successor.

Expanded polytetrafluoroethylene (e-PTFE)   Characterized as a porous teflon polymer with high stability in biologic systems. It is well tolerated, bioinert, resists breakdown by host tissues and by microbes, and does not elicit immunologic reactions.[22]   See also: *Expanded polytetrafluoroethylene (e-PTFE) membrane; Polytetrafluoroethylene (PTFE).*

Expanded polytetrafluoroethylene (e-PTFE) membrane   Barrier membrane made of a polymer of tetrafluoroethylene. e-PTFE is a matrix of polytetrafluoroethylene (PTFE) nodes and fibrils in a microstructure that can be varied in porosity to address the clinical and biologic requirements of its intended applications. Recognized for its inertness and tissue compatibility, e-PTFE is used to make several medical products, including e-PTFE membranes in a variety of shapes and sizes, in both nonreinforced and titanium-reinforced configurations. Titanium-reinforced configurations create more space and better maintain shape than nonreinforced configurations. This was the first type of membrane used in demonstrating the principle of guided bone regeneration (GBR). Widespread application established it as the standard for bone regeneration. However, clinical shortcomings, such as potential postoperative complications following membrane exposure and subsequent infection, or the obligatory second surgical procedure for membrane removal, have led to the development of bioresorbable membranes as alternatives.   See also: *Expanded polytetrafluoroethylene (e-PTFE).*

Experimental study   Study in which measurements are made to one independent variable while everything else around that one variable remains constant.[23]

Expert witness   Person qualified by the court to possess special knowledge, skill, or experience (scientific, technical, or other) and who can testify as an expert in a specific field. Expert witnesses can give opinions based on their special knowledge.

Exposure   Postoperative condition in which a membrane and/or implant is not covered by soft tissue because of wound dehiscence.

External abutment connection   Interface between a transmucosal component (abutment) and the coronal surface of an implant. The implant's coronal surface may have an external hexagon, which is engaged when the transmucosal component is seated.   See also: *Abutment connection.*[24,25]

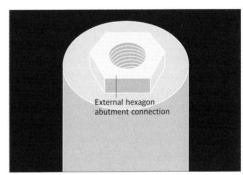

External abutment connection.

External bevel incision   Reduces the thickness of the mucogingival complex from the outside surface. Made from apical to coronal direction, it is used in gingivectomy procedures. Compare: *Internal bevel incision; Sulcular incision*.

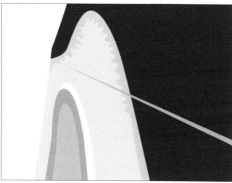

External bevel incision.
(Redrawn from Sato[26] with permission.)

External hexagon abutment connection   See: *External abutment connection; Hex*.

External hex implant
See: *External abutment connection; Hex*.

External irrigation   Application of physiologic saline solution during bone preparation for implant placement. It is provided by an external irrigation tube that is attached to the contra-angle handpiece.

Extracellular matrix (ECM)   (pl: *extracellular matrices (ECMS)*)   Material produced by cells and excreted to the extracellular space within the tissues. It takes the form of both ground substance and fibers and is composed chiefly of fibrous elements, proteins involved in cell adhesion, glycosaminoglycans, and other space-filling molecules. It serves as a scaffolding for holding tissues together, and its form and composition help determine tissue characteristics. The matrix may be mineralized to resist compression (as in bone) or dominated by tension-resisting fibers (as in tendon).

Extraction   Removal of a tooth or teeth.

Extraction socket   Open socket in the alveolar process following removal of a tooth.

Extraction socket graft   See: *Bio-Col technique*.

Extraosseous distractor   Jack-like device attached lateral to maxillary or mandibular basal bone for the purpose of creating incremental separation between jaw segments planned for distraction.[6]   See also: *Distraction osteogenesis (DO)*.

Extraoral graft   Graft harvested from extraoral sources, such as the calvarium, iliac crest, or tibia.

Exudate   Fluid filtered from the circulatory system into areas of inflammation. It contains proteins, solutes, and blood cells and results from the increased permeability of blood vessels caused by an inflammatory process. Pus, on the other hand, is characterized by the presence of bacteria and high concentrations of white blood cells. *Transudate*, also different from exudate, is fluid resulting from a disregulation of hydrostatic or osmotic pressure and is not a result of inflammation.

Eye prosthesis   See: *Exenteration*.

F

Facebow   Instrument used to record the positional relationship in the patient of the maxillary arch to the horizontal condylar axis of the mandible and to transfer this record to an articulating device that can simulate mandibular movements. A refinement to the conventional face-bow is known as a *kinematic* (hinge-bow) type, which has adjustable condylar rods, allowing the accurate location of the horizontal axis of mandibular rotation.[1,2]

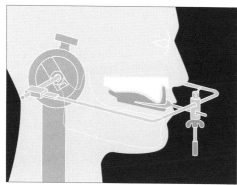

Facebow transfer to articulator.
(Redrawn from Sharry[3] with permission.)

Facial   Surface of incisors or canines and associated oral structures adjacent to the lips or cheeks.[4]

Facial moulage   Impression of facial soft tissues and bony contours to obtain a working cast for the fabrication of an extraoral prosthesis.[5]

Facial profile   Sagittal outline form of the face seen in the median plane.[4]

Facial prosthesis   Maxillofacial artificial replacement for a part of the face missing because of surgical, traumatic, or congenital etiology.   See also: *Craniofacial prosthesis; Maxillofacial prosthetics.*[4]

Facial symmetry   Mutually balanced relationship of facial parts relative to size, arrangement, or measurements.[6]

Facing   Tooth-colored material used to restore the visible surface of a prepared tooth or prosthetic replacement.[4]   See also: *Veneer*.

Fatigue   Property of metals that become embrittled and prone to fracture; caused by grain growth through repeated loading or flexure.

FDBA   Abbreviation for *Freeze-dried bone allograft*.

FEA   Abbreviation for *Finite element analysis*.

Fenestration   Buccal or lingual window defect of either bone or soft tissue, occurring over a tooth root, implant, or alveolar ridge.   See also: *Dehiscence*.

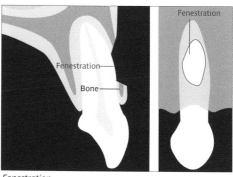

Fenestration.

Festoon   Contour of the soft tissues covering the roots of the teeth that tends to follow the cervical lines. Specifically in prosthodontics, a carving in the base material of a denture that simulates the contours of the natural tissues being replaced by the denture.

FGF   Abbreviation for *Fibroblast growth factor.*

FHA   Abbreviation for *Fluorohydroxyapatite.*

Fibrin clot   Clump that results from coagulation of the blood after a sequential process by which the multiple coagulation factors of the blood interact in the coagulation cascade. Essentially composed of fibrin, this insoluble protein is formed from fibrinogen by the proteolytic action of thrombin. Called also *blood clot.*

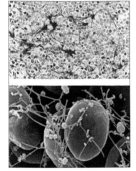

Fibrin clot (scanning electron micrographs; high magnification). (Reprinted from Lang et al[7] with permission.)

Fibrinolysis   (pl: *fibrinolyses*)   Enzymatic process of dissolution of fibrin. Plasmin, the main enzyme involved, degradates the fibrin mesh, leading to the production of circulating fragments that are cleared by other proteinases or organs.

Fibrin-rich matrix   Provisional matrix provided by the fibrin clot and fibronectin at the first phase of wound healing. It helps monocytes, fibroblasts, and epidermal cells migrate into the healing area.[8]

Fibroblast   Cell derived from mesoderm, predominant in the connective tissue. This flat elongated cell, with cytoplasmic processes at each end and a large, oval, vesicular nucleus, secretes fibrillar procollagen, fibronectin, and collagenase and is involved in extracellular matrix production and remodeling.

Fibroblast growth factor (FGF)   Family of growth factors with mitogenic properties for fibroblasts and mesoderm-derived cell types. They have important roles in angiogenesis, neurogenesis, wound healing, and tumor growth. In humans, more than 20 proteins have been identified as members of the FGF family. FGF-2, or basic FGF (bFGF), has been the most studied member of the FGF family for therapeutic purposes in regenerative treatments, notably soft tissue healing.

Fibromatosis   (pl: *fibromatoses*)   Group of tumor-like lesions that have an infiltrative nature and can be locally aggressive, making them difficult to remove completely. They can recur following surgery but do not metastasize to other parts of the body. Fibromatoses have also been known to undergo spontaneous regression and completely disappear.

Fibronectin   Adhesive glycoprotein with a high molecular weight (450 kd), composed of two disulfide-linked polypeptides. Functional domains of the molecule have an affinity for cells and the extracellular matrix components. It is found on cell surfaces, in connective tissues, in the blood, and in other body fluids. Fibronectins are important in connective tissue, where they cross-link to collagen, promote cellular adhesion and/or migration, and are involved in aggregation of platelets.

Fibrosseous integration   Direct attachment of bone to fibrous tissue without a definable intervening tissue.[9,10]   Compare: *Osseointegration.*

Fibrous   Property of being composed of, containing, or resembling fibers.

Fibrous connective tissue   Type of connective tissue that has a relatively high tensile strength because of a relatively high concentration of collagenous fibers. Such tissues form ligaments and tendons and are primarily composed of polysaccharides, proteins, and water. Called also *dense connective tissue.*

Fibrous encapsulation   Intervening growth of fibrous connective tissue between an endosseous implant and bone.[11]   See also: *Fibrosseous integration.*

Fibrous integration of implant   Interposition of healthy dense collagenous tissue between implant and bone.   See also: *Fibrous encapsulation.*

Fibula free flap   Graft used in oral and maxillofacial surgery for jaw reconstruction following tumor resection. It provides a long segment of bone and can include a large fasciocutaneous component. Flap harvested as osteocutaneous or purely osseous.

Fibular bone graft with free flap
See: *Fibula free flap.*

Finger-joint replacement   Artificial replacement for human finger joints, including the thumb.

Finite element analysis (FEA)   Science of creating computer simulations of mechanical or clinical situations. It is used to predict properties of structures and for structural design.

Finite element model   Structural simulation generated by computer programming.

First-stage surgery   See: *Stage-one surgery.*

Fisher exact test   Statistical test used in medical research, testing independence of rows and columns in a 2 x 2 contingency table (with 2 horizontal rows crossing 2 vertical columns, creating 4 places for data) based on exact sampling distribution of observed frequen-

cies. It was devised by British geneticist and biostatistician R. A. Fisher (1890 – 1962).[12,13]

Fistula   Abnormal connection between two anatomic cavities or an anatomic cavity and the external body surface. They can form as a result of trauma, infection, or inflammation.

Fixation, bicortical   See: *Bicortical stabilization.*

Fixation period   See: *Consolidation period.*

Fixation screw   Type of attachment screw used to secure a prosthetic component.[14] See also: *Attachment screw.*

Fixation tack   Element designed to resemble a simple tack. It is used to retain a membrane over augmentation material during ridge augmentation surgery.

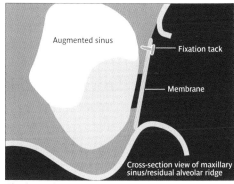

Fixation tack.

Fixed hybrid prosthesis   Nonremovable hybrid prosthesis.   See also: *Hybrid prosthesis.*

Fixed partial denture   Nonremovable partial prosthesis supported by teeth and/or implants.   See also: *Fixed prosthesis.*

Fixed prosthesis   Dental or maxillofacial prosthesis supported and retained by natural teeth, tooth roots, or dental implants, not readily removed by the patient. Synonym for *bridge.* See also: *Hybrid prosthesis; Implant-supported prosthesis (ISP); Provisional prosthesis.*

Fixture Term used in early Brånemark literature to refer to an implant.[11] See also: *Endosseous implant*.

Flap Soft tissue that is raised or elevated for surgical access. See also: *Envelope flap; Mucoperiosteal flap; Partial-thickness flap*.

> **Apically positioned f.** Surgical flap that is moved apically to a new position.

> **Coronally positioned f.** Surgical flap that is moved to a new position coronal to its previous position.

Flapless surgery Implant placement performed without the elevation of a flap.

Fleece, collagen See: *Collagen fleece*.

Fluoride-modifying surface treatment Implant treatment that exposes the surface to a cleansing bath of hydrofluoric acid following treatment with etching or blasting. This technique has been shown to improve biomechanical anchorage and bone integration when compared to control implants treated without the hydrofluoric acid bath.

Fluorochrome Fluorescent substance used as a stain or label for biologic specimens. In implant dentistry, it is used in research to evaluate the kinetics of osteogenesis and osseointegration on implant surfaces.

Fluorohydroxyapatite (FHA) Pyrolytical segmentation of natural algae and hydrothermal transformation of the calcium carbonate ($CaCO_3$) skeleton of algae into FHA ($Ca5(PO_4)3OHxF^{1-x}$). Particles consist of a pore system (mean diameter 10 µm), periodically septated (mean interval 30 µm) and interconnectively microperforated (mean diameter of perforations 1 µm).

Fluorosis Condition that occurs because of excessive intake of fluoride either through naturally occurring fluoride in the water, water fluoridation, toothpaste, or other sources. Damage in tooth development from the overexposure to fluoride typically occurs between the ages of 6 months and 5 years. Teeth are generally composed of hydroxyapatite and carbonated hydroxyapatite, and when fluoride is present, fluorapatite is created. Excessive fluoride can cause yellowing of teeth, white spots, and pitting or mottling of enamel, and the teeth become hypocalcified. Although it is usually the permanent teeth that are affected, occasionally primary teeth may be involved. In mild cases, there may be a few white flecks or small pits on the enamel of the teeth. In more severe cases, there may be brown stains. Differential diagnosis for this condition may include Turner hypoplasia (although this is usually more localized), some mild forms of amelogenesis imperfecta, and other environmental enamel defects of diffuse and demarcated opacities.

Follow-up Periodic monitoring of patient health after medical or surgical treatment, including that of clinical study or trial participants.[12]

Food and Drug Administration (FDA) Agency of United States Department of Health and Human Services that regulates testing of experimental drugs and devices. The FDA clears new drugs and medical products based on evidence of safety and efficacy.

Force Vector of load application creating acceleration or deformation along the direction of its application. See also: *Biting force; Closure force; Distribution force; Pullout force*.

> **Axial f.** Force directed axially or through the long axis of an object.

> **Lateral f.** In dentistry, forces other than axial in direction.

Force vector Force applied through direction and magnitude.

Fracture See: *Bone fracture.*

   Porcelain f. See: *Porcelain fracture.*

   Screw f. See: *Screw fracture.*

Framework Core component of implant prosthesis, generally fabricated of metallic or ceramic material and veneered with ceramic or resin coatings. It is incorporated in fixed prostheses for strength and retention of matrices and teeth. For removable prostheses, it can be designed to provide prosthesis retention, support, and stability.[4,15]

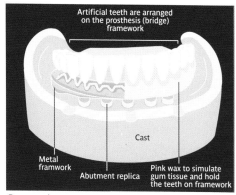

Framework.
(Redrawn from Taylor and Laney[16] with permission.)

Framework misfit Contacting surface discrepancy between an accurately fitting framework and one which does not fit accurately.

Free gingiva See: *Marginal gingiva.*

Free gingival graft Soft tissue graft taken from the patient's palate that includes the epithelium.

Free-standing implant Implant that is not connected to a natural tooth or other implants.

Freeze-dried bone allograft (FDBA) Most commonly used allograft, which is frozen and freeze-dried (lyophilized). It may form bone or participate in new bone formation by osteoinduction or osteoconduction. It is effective when used with barrier membranes. The freezing and freeze-drying process essentially lowers the antigenicity.

Freeze-drying Method of tissue preparation in which a tissue specimen is frozen and then dehydrated at a low temperature under high-vacuum conditions. In this process, the frozen water in material is sublimated directly from solid phase to gas. See also: *Lyophilization.*

Frenectomy Surgical excision of a frenulum, including its attachment to underlying bone, that is objectionable either functionally or esthetically. This procedure can be accomplished with a conventional blade or a carbon dioxide (CO_2) laser.[17] Called also *frenulectomy.*

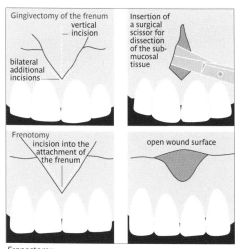

Frenectomy.
(Redrawn from Ito and Johnson[18] with permission.)

Frenotomy Incision of the frenulum.[17]

Frenulum (pl: *frenula*) Fold of mucous membrane, usually with enclosed muscle fibers, that attaches the lips and cheeks to alveolar mucosa and/or gingiva and underlying periosteum.[17] Called also *frenum*.

Friction-fit Component retained and/or stabilized through frictional contact with another component.

Front See: *Anterior.*

Full crown See: *Crown.*

Full-thickness flap See: *Mucoperiosteal flap.*

Full-thickness graft Gingival graft including the epithelium, connective tissue, and periosteum.

Functional ankylosis Concept developed by Andre Schroeder in 1981 to describe the junction between an implant and surrounding bone. Elasticity of bone makes contact and connection a functional unit in which contact between implant and bone is maintained.[19] See also: *Osseointegration.*

Functional loading Load applied to teeth or implant-supported prosthesis during normal chewing function.

Fusobacterium nucleatum Gram-negative, nonmotile, anaerobic, rod-shaped bacterium commonly associated with periodontal and peri-implant disease.

G

Gamma-linolenic acid (GLA) protein
See: *Osteocalcin.*

Gamma ray   Part of electromagnetic radiation with the smallest wavelengths and thus the most energy of any wave in the electromagnetic spectrum.

Gap   See: *Edentulous space.*

GBR   Abbreviation for *Guided bone regeneration.*

GCF   Abbreviation for *Gingival crevicular fluid.*

Gene therapy   Treatment of human disease by the transfer of genetic material into specific cells.[1]

   Nonviral g. t.   Method of gene therapy that uses nonviral vectors to deliver genetic material into target cells, ie, plasmid DNA and synthetic vectors (eg, lipoplexes, polyplexes).

   Viral g. t.   Method of gene therapy that uses viruses as gene-delivery vectors; viruses have a portion of their genome replaced by a therapeutic gene. The most widely used viruses are adenovirus, adeno-associated virus, lentivirus, and retrovirus.

Gene transfer   Introduction of genes into cells. The viral particle binds to specific cellular receptors and is taken up by endocytosis. Acidification of the endosome results in release to the cytoplasm and partial disassembly of the viral particle. Transport through the nuclear pore is by viral proteins. Once in the nucleus the DNA remains extrachromosomal, and transcription and translation are by the host cell's own protein synthetic machinery.   See also: *Gene therapy.*

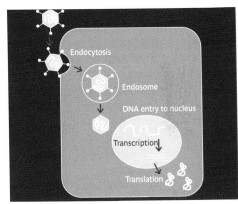

Gene transfer by an adenovirus vector.
(Redrawn from Partridge and Oreffo[2] with permission.)

Gingiva   (pl: *gingivae*)   That part of the masticatory mucosa covering the alveolar process and surrounding cervical portion of teeth. This fibrous connective tissue, covered by keratinized epithelium, is contiguous with periodontal ligament and mucosal tissues of the mouth.[3]   See also: *Attached gingiva; Keratinized gingiva; Marginal gingiva.*

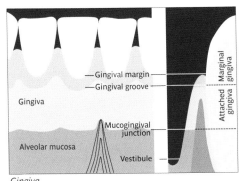

Gingiva.
(Redrawn from Genco et al[4] with permission.)

Free g. See: *Marginal gingiva.*

Gingival abscess Localized purulent infection involving the marginal gingivae or interdental papillae.[5]

Gingival cleft Vertical fissure in gingiva occurring over a dehiscence of bone covering a root.

Gingival crater Saucer-shaped defect of interproximal gingiva.[5]

Gingival crevice See: *Gingival sulcus.*

Gingival crevicular fluid (GCF) Serum ultrafiltrate tissue fluid that seeps into the gingival sulcus from gingival connective tissue and vasculature through thin sulcular epithelia. GCF is increased in the presence of inflammation and contains multiple mediators involved in inflammation, connective tissue homeostasis, and host response.

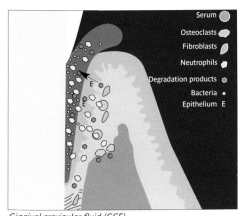

Gingival crevicular fluid (GCF).
(Reprinted from Uitto[6] with permission.)

Gingival curettage Process of debriding the soft tissue wall of a periodontal pocket.[5]

Gingival disease See: *Gingivitis; Periodontal disease; Periodontitis.*

Gingival enlargement Increase in size of the gingiva. Gingival enlargement may result from systemic drug use. Drugs commonly associated with this condition include calcium channel blockers, cyclosporin, and dilantin. Called also *gingival overgrowth.*[7]

Gingival epithelium See: *Epithelium.*

Gingival graft Autogenous graft of masticatory mucosa or collagenous tissue completely or partially detached from its original site and placed in a prepared recipient bed. See also: *Free gingival graft.*

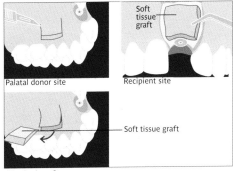

Gingival graft.
(Redrawn from Langer[8] with permission.)

Gingival hyperplasia Enlargement of the gingiva associated with increase in number of cells, typically connective tissue-derived cells.

Gingival hypertrophy Enlargement of the gingiva because of increase in size of cells.

Gingival margin See: *Marginal gingiva.*

Gingival overgrowth See: *Gingival enlargement.*

Gingival papilla Portion of the gingiva that occupies interproximal spaces; interdental or interimplant extension of the gingiva.

Gingival recession Location of gingival margin apical to the cementoenamel junction or implant connection. Marginal tissue recessions were classified by Miller in four classes according to predictability of root coverage. *Class I:* recession does not extend to the mucogingival junction and there is no tissue loss in the interproximal area. *Class II:* recession extends to or beyond the mucogingival junction. There is no periodontal loss in the interproximal area. *Class III:* recession extends to or beyond the mucogingival junction. Bone or soft tissue loss is present in the interdental area, or there is malpositioning of the teeth which prevents total root coverage. *Class IV:* recession extends to or beyond the mucogingival junction. The bone or soft tissue loss in the interdental area and/or malpositioning of teeth is so severe that root coverage cannot be anticipated.

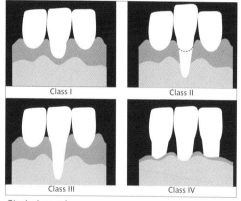

Gingival recession.
(Redrawn from Miller[9] with permission.)

Gingival stippling Pitted, orange-peel appearance frequently seen in attached gingiva. Although it is commonly seen in healthy gingiva, it is not a requirement for gingival health.

Gingival sulcus Shallow space coronal to attachment of the junctional epithelium. It is bound by tooth and sulcular epithelium on either side. The coronal extent of gingival sulcus is the gingival margin. Called also *gingival crevice.*

Gingivectomy Excision of a portion of the gingiva, usually performed to reduce soft tissue wall of periodontal pocket or to remove excess tissue in the condition of gingival enlargement. In the figure, the spots are marks on the outer aspect of the gingiva to delineate the bottom of the pocket and indicate incision design.

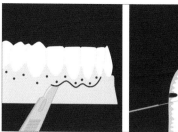

Gingivectomy.
(Redrawn from Lindhe et al[10] with permission.)

Gingivitis Inflammation of the gingiva. See also: *Periodontitis.*

Gingivoplasty Surgical reshaping of the gingiva.

Gingivostomatitis (pl: *gingivostomatitides*) Inflammation and ulcers affecting both the gingiva and the oral mucosa. The condition typically is the result of a viral infection.

GLA protein Abbreviation for *gamma-linolenic acid protein.* See: *Osteocalcin.*

Glass ceramic Ceramic of silicon dioxide or similar materials that solidify from molten state without crystallizing. See also: *Ceramic.*

Glucocorticoid Group of C21 steroid hormones (eg, cortisol) that affect carbohydrate, fat, and protein metabolism. They are secreted from the adrenal cortex and used in treatment of desquamative gingival lesions in the oral cavity. Called also *corticosteroid.*

Glucoprotein See: *Glycoprotein.*

Glycoprotein Conjugated protein in which the nonprotein group is generally a carbohydrate. It can contain one or more covalently linked carbohydrate residues. Called also *glucoprotein.*

Glycosaminoglycan Polysaccharide chain of hexosamine alternating with another carbohydrate residue. It is a component of proteoglycan, which is a major part of noncollagenous matrix of bone and connective tissues. Called also *mucopolysaccharide*.

Gnathology Division of the dental art and science concerned with the interrelationship of the biologic elements of the masticatory system in their occlusal static and functional states. These elements include the anatomy, histology, physiology, and pathology applicable to diagnosis and restorative treatment.[11,12]

Gold cylinder attachment Attachment element comprising part of a prosthetic component. This term specifically refers to the alloy used in fabrication of the element. Called also *cylinder-to-transmucosal element*.[13] See also: *Attachment element*.

Graft Organ tissue used for implantation or transplantation. Living tissue placed in contact with injured tissue to repair a defect or supply a deficiency. To induce union between normally separate tissues. Graft options may include both vital and nonvital materials. See also: *Allogeneic bone graft; Alloplast; Alloplastic graft; Autogenous bone graft; Block bone graft; Bone graft; Extraoral graft; Fibula free flap; Free gingival graft; Full-thickness graft; Gingival graft; Maxillary sinus floor graft; Nonvascularized free graft; One-stage grafting procedures; Onlay graft; Osteoconductive graft; Soft tissue augmentation; Subepithelial connective tissue graft; Two-stage grafting procedures; Xenograft.*

Graft healing The restoration of implanted living tissue to its original intergrity. Bone graft healing has two different routes: either it fails to incorporate and gradually disappears, or it becomes incorporated as a mechanically functioning part of the host bone. Osteoblasts or osteoprogenitor cells may be transferred to recipient site. Via resorption of bone graft, various growth factors are released from the noncollagenous part of bone matrix.

Granulation tissue Healing tissue consisting of fibroblasts, capillary buds, inflammatory cells, and edema.

Grit-blasted implant surface Modification of an implant or other surface through the application of sand, aluminum oxide, or other abrasive material by intense air pressure. See also: *Rough implant surface; Sandblasted implant surface.*

Group function Simultaneous working-side contact of primarily posterior teeth during lateral movements of the mandible for broad distribution of occlusal forces.[12]

Growth factor Diverse group of polypeptides with important roles in the regulation of growth and the development of a variety of organs. These factors control key aspects involved in wound repair, including cellular mitogenesis, matrix biosynthesis, chemotaxis, and differentiation. See also: *Cytokine; Fibroblast growth factor (FGF); Insulin-like growth factor (IGF); Plasma-containing growth factor; Platelet-derived growth factor (PDGF); Platelet-rich plasma (PRP); Transforming growth factor (TGF); Vascular endothelial growth factor (VEGF).*

Growth hormone Protein hormone of about 190 amino acids that is synthesized and secreted by cells called *somatotrophs* in the anterior pituitary. It is a major participant in control of several complex physiologic processes, including growth and metabolism.

GTR Abbreviation for *Guided tissue regeneration*.

Guide See: *Radiographic template; Stereolithographic guide, Surgical template.*

Guide pin   Type of laboratory screw used in the fabrication of a prosthetic restoration. Surgical or restorative adjunctive marker used to indicate implant angulation or location when preparing osteotomy sites.   See also: *Incisal guide pin.*

Guide stent   See: *Surgical template.*

Guided bone regeneration (GBR)   Follows the principle of maintaining a surgically created space at a bony defect via a barrier membrane, thus excluding rapidly proliferating epithelial cells and fibroblasts and permitting the growth of slower-growing bone cells and blood vessels. Graft material may also be used in combination with barrier membranes in GBR procedures to support the membrane and prevent its collapse. In addition, bone grafts provide a scaffold upon which new bone can form.   See also: *Alveolar ridge augmentation, Guided bone regeneration for; Bone regeneration.*

Guided tissue regeneration (GTR)   Surgical procedure aimed at regenerating lost periodontal attachment. Creation of a secluded space favoring angiogenic and osteogenic cells, protecting the vascular and cellular elements while probably supporting accumulation of growth factors. True periodontal regeneration must include new cementum formation, periodontal ligament, and alveolar bone on a previously diseased root surface. GTR follows the principle of maintaining a surgically created space around teeth via a barrier membrane, thus allowing the slower–proliferating periodontal ligament cells, bone cells, and possibly cementoblasts to populate the root surface. This term is not to be confused with *guided bone regeneration (GBR)*, which describes a similar principle for isolated bone defects following tooth loss and concerns the regeneration or augmentation of bone only.

Gypsum   See: *Medical-grade calcium sulfate.*

G

H

H   Abbreviation for *Hounsfield unit.*

HA   Abbreviation for *Hydroxyapatite.*

Hader bar   Rectangular bar with rounded occlusal ridge that rigidly connects teeth or implants and receives a plastic sleeve attachment for prosthesis retention.[1,2]   See also: *Clip bar overdenture.*

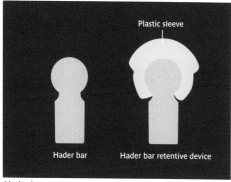

Hader bar.
(Redrawn from Preiskel[1] with permission.)

Hanau formula   See: *Hanau Quint.*

Hanau Quint   Five factors involved in developing a balanced articulation for removable complete dentures: incisal guidance, condylar guidance, cusp height, plane of occlusion, and compensating curve. First described by Rudolph Hanau in 1926 and incorporated in the design of a semi-adjustable articulator (Hanau H) that provided for horizontal condylar guidance to be set using an intraoral protrusive interocclusal record. Lateral condylar guidance (L) can then be calculated using the Hanau formula, L = H/8 + 12, where H is the recorded horizontal condylar guidance.[2,3]

Hand prosthesis   Artificial substitute for a human hand.

Harvest   Procurement of a graft from a donor site.

Haversian canal   See: *Osteon.*

Haversian system   See: *Osteon.*

Hazard ratio   The risk of an event occurring in one group compared with another when the primary response variable is the time to event. A hazard ratio of 1 indicates that neither group is more at risk for the event than the other. If the hazard ratio is, for example, 5, then one group is five times more likely to experience the event than the other.[4]

HBOT   Abbreviation for *Hyperbaric oxygen treatment.*

Healing   Process of cure; repair or regeneration of injured, lost, or surgically treated tissue.

Healing abutment   Implant component placed at stage-two surgery to guide periodontal soft tissue healing prior to definitive prosthetic restoration. Typical cross-sectional design is cylindrical. See also: *Anatomic healing abutment.* (See figure next page.)

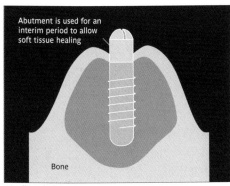

Abutment is used for an interim period to allow soft tissue healing

Bone

Healing abutment.

Healing by first intention   Restoration of continuity of wound edges directly by fibrous adhesion without intervention of granulations. Called also *healing by primary intention; primary adhesion; primary union.*

Healing by secondary intention   Wound closure wherein the edges of the wound remain separated, and healing occurs from the base and sides of the wound toward the surface via formation of granulation tissue. Called also *secondary adhesion; secondary union.*

Healing cap   See: *Healing abutment.*

Healing collar   See: *Healing abutment.*

Healing screw   Type of healing element. A covering screw to protect an implant and guide wound healing during the osseointegration process.   See also: *Healing abutment.*

Hearing aid   See: *Bone-anchored hearing aid (BAHA).*

Heat-curing resin   Resin requiring external heat to activate polymerization.

HEMA   Abbreviation for *hydroxyethylmethacrylate.*   See: *Alloplastic graft.*

Hematopoietic stem cell   Progenitor or precursor cells found in the bone marrow from which all blood cell types of both the myeloid and lymphoid lineages are derived.

Hemi-maxillectomy   Partial surgical removal of the maxilla.

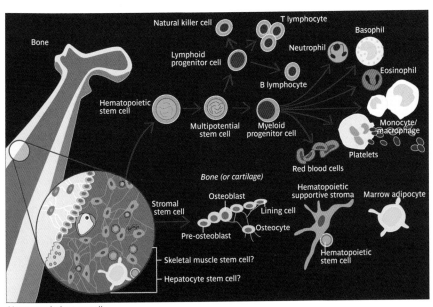

Hematopoietic stem cell.
(Redrawn from Winslow and Kibink[5] with permission.)

Hemorrhage   Bleeding, often excessive and may be uncontrollable.

Hemostasis   Control of bleeding, via either the patient's intrinsic clotting ability or clinical measures taken to assist the process.

Heterogenous graft   See: *Xenograft.*

Heterograft   See: *Xenograft.*

Hex   Implant design featuring a six-sided implant-abutment interface.[6,7]

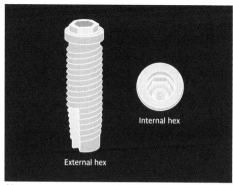

Internal hex

External hex

Hex.

Histomorphometry   Method of quantifying and analyzing structures, eg, bone, soft tissue, and vascularity, from histologic specimens; involves a large range of measurements, including numbers, length, surface area, volume, angles, and curvature.

Hole   See: *Access hole.*

Hollow cylinder   See: *Implant basket.*

Homograft   See: *Allogeneic bone graft.*

Homologous graft   See: *Allogeneic bone graft.*

Horizontal osteotomy   Horizontal surgical cut in bone.

Host response   Defense mechanism triggered in graft recipient, often by pathogenic stimuli (eg, bacteria from the dental biofilm).

Hounsfield unit (H)   Value on a quantitative scale indicating the degree of attenuation of x-rays by tissue in computerized tomography (CT) and thus describing radiodensity of the tissue. The name was given in honor of Godfrey N. Hounsfield, who presented the first CT scanner in 1972.

Howship lacuna   Small pit or groove formed by resorbing osteoclasts on the surface of bone undergoing resorption.   See also: *Osteoclast.*

Hybrid prosthesis   Fixed, removable, or maxillofacial prosthesis designed and fabricated with an atypical combination of materials or structural components.[8]

Hydroxyapatite (HA)   Bone substitute, $Ca_{10}(PO_4)6(OH)_2$, which may be ceramic or nonceramic. The ceramic form is manufactured by a sintering process, in which the HA is heated to 1100°C, whereby the crystals fuse and grow in size.   See also: *Bovine-derived anorganic bone matrix; Hydroxyapatite implant surface; Porous coralline hydroxyapatite; Porous marine-derived coralline hydroxyapatite.*

Hydroxyapatite-bone grafting   Method of grafting in which granules of hydroxyapatite can be added to chips of autogenous bone to obtain the desired shape and compromise or delay resorption.

Hydroxyapatite implant surface   Primarily insoluble or partially soluble amorphous and crystalline calcium phosphate coating applied to the surface of an implant, intended to enhance osseointegration.

H

Hydroxyethylmethacrylate (HEMA)
See: *Alloplastic graft.*

Hygiene cap   See: *Healing abutment.*

Hyperalgesia   Increased pain response to a normally painful stimulus.

Hyperbaric oxygen treatment (HBOT)   Therapy used in irradiated cancer patients to improve wound healing and osseointegration of implants. Administration of 100% oxygen under increased atmospheric pressure (usually 2 atm or 10 m sea water). The elevated partial pressure of oxygen to tissues has been shown to improve angiogenesis, bone metabolism, and success of osseointegration. It has been recommended that patients receive several treatments in a hyperbaric oxygen chamber, both pre- and postoperatively. This therapy also has been used to treat severe anaerobic infections in the jaws.[9]

Hyperesthesia   Increased sensitivity to noxious or non-noxious stimuli.

Hyperocclusion   Premature or abnormal contact of opposing teeth, creating excessive or traumatic force.[10]

Hyperparathyroidism   Physical condition created by excessive amounts of parathyroid hormone. *Primary hyperparathyroidism* is caused by the dysfunction of the parathyroid glands. This results in oversecretion of the parathyroid hormone (PTH), leading to increased bone resorption and subsequent hypercalcemia, as well as reduced renal clearance of calcium and increased intestinal calcium absorption. *Secondary hyperparathyroidism* is usually the result of chronic renal failure and resistance to the action of PTH. Hyperparathyroidism was previously thought to be associated with loss of radicular lamina dura and brown tumors of the bone; however, a recent study in the contemporary population of patients indicated that changes are much more subtle and include anticipated reductions in cortical bone but do not appear to have a significant impact on periodontal health. New findings such as increased incidence of oral tori may reflect a form of anabolic action of PTH in bone.[11]

Hyperplasia   (pl: *hyperplasias*)   Abnormal multiplication or increase in number of normal cells, resulting in an increase in tissue mass or organ size. To be distinguished from *hypertrophy*, which is related to an increase in cell size.

Hypertension   Persistent, sustained high blood pressure of 140/90 mm Hg or above. Hypertension becomes a surgical risk factor if the condition is uncontrolled.

Hypertrophy   Non-tumor-associated increase in tissue or organ size related to an increase in constituent cell size. A hypertrophic response may occur as a result of a particular condition. To be distinguished from *hyperplasia*, which is related to an increase in cell number.

Hypoesthesia   Decreased perception of stimulation by noxious or non-noxious stimuli.

I

I-beam principle   See: *Moment of inertia.*

ICTP   Abbreviation for *C-terminal telopeptide of type I collagen*.   See: *C-telopeptide pyridinoline cross-links of type I collagen.*

IGF   Abbreviation for *Insulin-like growth factor*.

IIL   Abbreviation for *Interleukin*.

Iliac bone   See: *Ilium.*

Iliac crest   Long, curved superior border of the ilium. Serves as a donor site for most preferred autogenous grafts for larger augmentation procedures.[1]   See also: *Iliac crest graft; Ilium.*

Iliac crest graft   Common extraoral cortico-cancellous autogenous bone graft used in cases where large block volumes for alveolar ridge reconstruction are required.   See also: *Alveolar ridge augmentation; Iliac bone grafting for.*

Ilium   The largest and uppermost portion of hip bone. The hip bone is the broadest bone of the skeleton, located in the sidewall and anterior wall of the pelvis. It is made up of three bones or parts: the ilium, ischium, and pubis.

Image guidance   General technique of using preoperative diagnostic imaging with computer-based planning tools to facilitate surgical and restorative plans and procedures.[2-4]

Imaging guide   Scan to determine bone volume, inclination and shape of the alveolar process, and bone height and width, which is used at surgical site.   See also: *Computed tomography (CT) scan; Three-dimensional guidance system for implant placement; Backscattered electron (BSE) imaging.*

Immediate functional loading   Implant prosthesis is seated at the time of implant placement and immediately subjected to functional loading.   See also: *Functional loading.*

Immediate implant placement   Implant placement immediately following extraction of a tooth. This procedure must be combined in most patients with a bone-grafting technique to eliminate peri-implant bone defects.

Immediate loading   Application of functional or nonfunctional load to an implant at the time of surgical placement or shortly thereafter; generally considered to be loading within 48 hours of implant placement.[5]   See also: *Immediate functional loading; Immediate nonfunctional loading.*

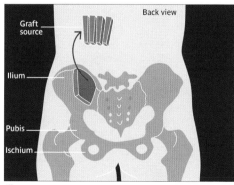

Ilium.

Orthodontics and i. l. Loading of temporary orthodontic implants immediately after placement, without an intervening period of unloaded healing. See also: *Orthodontic anchorage implant.*

Tooth extraction and i. l. Implant placed and put into function at the time the natural tooth is extracted.

Immediate nonfunctional loading Implant prosthesis is seated at the time of implant placement but kept out of direct occlusal contact. Loading occurs from lip and tongue pressure and contact with food, but not from contact with the opposing teeth.

Immediate provisionalization Fabrication and seating of provisional restoration at time of implant placement. The provisional restoration may or may not be designed for immediate functional occlusal contact.[6]

Immediate restoration Dental prosthesis placed immediately following the removal of a natural tooth or teeth.[7,8] See: *Immediate provisionalization.*

Immunity Condition of being immune; all mechanisms used by the body as protection against foreign environmental agents. See also: *Acquired immunity; Innate immunity.*

Immunocompetence Ability or capacity to develop a normal immune response following exposure to antigen.

Immunoglobulin Glycoprotein composed of heavy and light peptide chains; functions as antibody in serum and secretions. There are five major classes (IgG, IgA, IgM, IgE, and IgD) on the basis of structure and biologic activity.

Immunologic response Bodily defense in reaction to an invading substance (antigen, such as virus, fungus, bacteria, or transplanted organ) that produces a response, including antibody production, cell-mediated immunity, or immunologic tolerance.

Impaction of tooth Developmental disturbance in which a tooth does not fully erupt into occlusion. It may be a tooth bud or fully developed tooth surrounded by bone, either partially or fully. The most frequently impacted teeth are mandibular third molars.

Implant Biocompatible alloplastic device, tissue, or substance surgically placed into recipient for the improvement of an existing condition. Generally placed for restorative purposes but may also be used with diagnostic or experimental intentions.[7,9] See also: *Angled/angulated implant; Blade implant; Complete subperiosteal implant; Craniofacial implant; Cylindrical implant; Disk implant; Distraction implant; Endosseous implant; Endosseous ramus implant; Eposteal implant; Free-standing implant; Malpositioned implant; Mini-implant; Nonsubmerged implant; Nonthreaded implant; Ocular implant; One-piece implant; Percutaneous implant; Provisional implant; Ramus frame implant; Root-form implant; Skin-penetrating implant; Sleeper implant; Tapered implant; Threaded implant; Transosseous implant; Two-piece implant; Zygomatic implant.*

Implant abutment See: *Abutment; Angled/angulated abutment; CAD/CAM abutment; Ceramic abutment; Castable abutment; Nonangled abutment; Nonrotating abutment; Transmucosal abutment.*

Implant-abutment interface Surface forming a common boundary between the abutment and implant.[10] See also: *Microgap.*

Implant anchorage Use of endosseous implant for anchorage during tooth movement in orthodontic treatment. Used to provide resistance to unwanted natural tooth movement. Also, use of implants in orthodontic treatment to provide anchorage for prosthesis.[11]

Implant axis   Axis through the body of an implant dictated by its greatest dimension.

Implant basket   Design feature of an implant that has a hollow apical portion, which allows a core of bone to remain in the preparation of the osteotomy site and fit within the confines of the hollow apical portion. Called also *inverted basket* or *hollow cylinder*.[12,13]

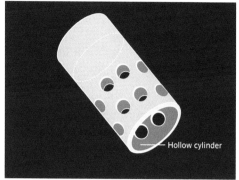

Implant basket.

Implant body   Anchorage component embedded in tissue, usually bone, by which all other components in an implant system are supported. Other components are stacked or threaded one into another.[14]

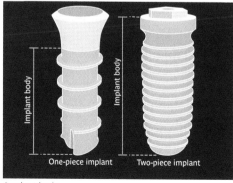

Implant body.

Implant-bone interface   When bone substitutes are applied, newly formed host bone creates an interface between the implant surface and alveolar bone as the implant becomes osseointegrated.

Implant collar   Most coronal portion of an implant or anchorage component. The collar can have the same surface finish as the remaining portion of the implant anchorage component or have a different surface finish designed by a manufacturer.

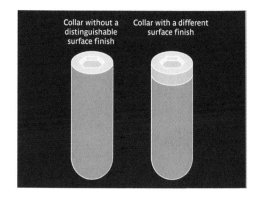

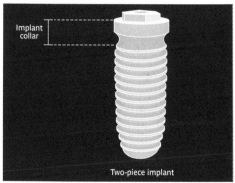

Implant collar.

Implant component   "One of the principal portions of an implant system or one of the structural sections of a dental implant abutment."[15,16]

Implant configuration   Pattern or arrangement of the positions of two or more implants placed intraorally.

Implant-crown ratio   See: *Crown-implant ratio*.

Implant dentistry   Field of dental art and science concerned with diagnosis and treatment planning for implant–supported restorations, surgical placement of implants, and the

Implant design   Conceptualization of an implant form at the planning or designing stage as carried through production.

Implant diameter   Length of the horizontal axis through the center of an implant body. Anchorage components (implants) are available in various diameters and lengths, and the dimensions vary among the various implant manufacturers. The symbol used to reflect the diameter is Ø.

Implant exposure   Postoperative condition in which an implant is not completely covered by soft tissues because of wound dehiscence. A second surgical procedure following implant placement is used to access the implant shoulder, remove the healing screw, and replace it with an abutment. This can be accomplished with a punch technique or flap elevation.

Implant head   Most coronal part or area of an implant. The same area, ie the coronal surface, can be referred to as the *platform*.

Implant insertion   See: *Implant placement.*

Implant installation   See: *Implant placement.*

Implant interface   Contacting surface of living tissue (bone) and nonliving alloplast (implant).[6,7]   See also: *Osseointegration.*

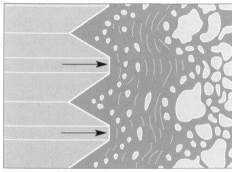

Implant interface (arrows).
(Redrawn from Brånemark et al[17] with permission.)

Implant length   Straight-line dimension of the vertical axis of an implant body. Anchorage components (implants) available in various diameters and lengths. Dimensions vary for specific applications among the various implant manufacturers.

Implant-level impression   To record an implant platform at the tissue level, a coping is attached to the implant and an impression is made for laboratory restorative procedures. The resultant cast usually contains an elastomeric material at the implant site.[6]

Implant loading   Act of placing forces on an implant through function and/or parafunction.   See also: *Delayed loading; Dynamic loading; Early loading; Immediate functional loading; Immediate nonfunctional loading; Static loading.*

Alveolar bone growth and i. l.   Phenomenon observed beneath mandibular cantilever prostheses. Considered to be an example of Wolff Law of bone loading.[18]

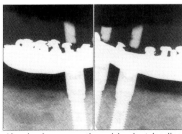

Alveolar bone growth and implant loading (prosthesis placement).

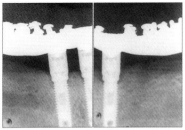

Alveolar bone growth and implant loading (2 years, 8 months; increase in crestal bone height: 3mm).

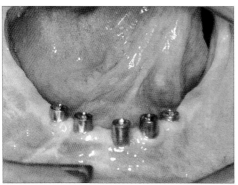

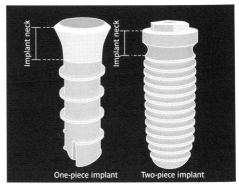

Alveolar bone growth and implant loading (2 years, 8 months; osseous proliferation). (Reprinted from Taylor[18] with permission.)

Implant neck.

Implant loss   Circumstances whereby the implant is removed from the patient.   See also: *Early implant loss; Late implant loss.*

Implant material   See: *Commercially pure titanium (CPTi); Hydroxyapatite (HA); Titanium alloy; Zirconium oxide.*

Implant micromotion, effects of
See: *Micromotion.*

Implant micromovement   Relative motion between an implant body and its investing tissues at the microscopic level; not clinically visible.

Implant mobility   Relative motion between an implant body and its investing tissues.

Implant mount   Component positioned onto the implant facilitating surgical placement of the implant into the osteotomy site. May be removed by loosening the attachment mechanism to the implant, either through removal of a screw or release of a frictional fit into the implant.[14,19]

Implant neck   Coronal portion of the implant in which a constriction in diameter width may or may not be present below the platform area.[20]   See also: *Cervix; Implant collar.*

Implant osseointegration   See: *Osseointegration.*

Implant overdenture   Complete or partial removable prosthesis that covers and is supported by dental implants, individual or splinted, and related tissue structures.[6]

Bar-clip attachment and i. o.   Removable prosthesis covering and supported by endosseous implants. The implants are connected by a bar, and support is provided by associated hard and soft tissue structures. The overdenture receives its retention in part by a clip embedded in the impression surface of the acrylic resin base.   See also: *Denture.*

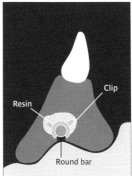

Bar-clip attachment and implant overdenture (in cross section). (Redrawn from Brudvik[21] with permission.)

Implant periapical lesion   Rarely seen radiolucency at the apex of dental implants that can lead to fistula formation. It has been speculated that these osteolytic lesions may be caused by residual bacteria in the bony recipient site.[22]

Implant placement   Surgical procedure for the placement of a dental implant in bone.   See also: *Early implant placement; Immediate implant placement; Late implant placement; One-stage grafting procedures; Two-stage grafting procedures.*

> **Bone grafting and i. p.**   See: *Guided bone regeneration (GBR); Maxillary sinus floor elevation.*

Implant placement, after extraction
See: *Immediate implant placement.*

Implant placement, in irradiated bone   Irradiated cancer patients are at higher risk for the failure of achieving osseointegration. However, the use of long implants, fixed retention, and adjuvant hyperbaric oxygen therapy has resulted in a decrease of implant failures. Clearly, the clinician and patient should be aware of the considerations involving irradiated patients, and a team approach should be applied.[23]

Implant placement, with maxillary sinus floor elevation   Implants may be placed simultaneously with a sinus floor elevation when the residual bone height is sufficient for primary implant stability. Otherwise, a staged approach must be considered.   See also: *Maxillary sinus floor elevation.*

Implant prosthesis   See: *Implant-supported prosthesis (ISP).*

Implant prosthodontics   Subspecialty area of prosthodontics concerned with the replacement of missing natural teeth and associated tissues with restorations supported by dental implants.[7]   See also: *Implant dentistry.*

Implant pullout strength   See: *Pullout strength.*

Implant reopening   See: *Implant exposure.*

Implant retention   Resistance to displacement (vertically) in the plane of placement. Dental implant(s) may be used for prosthesis retention alone or as part of a coupling system providing retention, support, and stability for the prosthesis. Rarely could implants provide retention only without simultaneously providing some degree of prosthesis stability as well.

Implant shaft   Portion of the implant between the coronal and apical ends.   See also: *Implant body.*

Implant shape   Design used to categorize the type of implant, such as cylinder, blade, frame, or button.[24]

Implant shoulder position   Final apicocoronal position of the implant shoulder, as determined by the surgeon, relative to the alveolar crest, ie, supracrestal, crestal, or subcrestal.

> **I. s. p., Crestal**   At the level of the bony ridge crest.

> **I. s. p., Subcrestal**   Below the level of the bony ridge crest. (See figure next page.)

> **I. s. p., Supracrestal**   Above the level of the bony ridge crest. (See figure next page.)

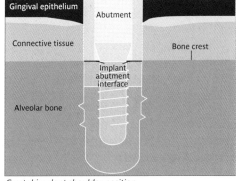

Crestal implant shoulder position.

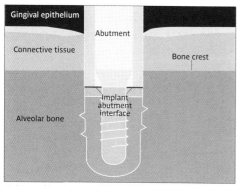

Subcrestal implant shoulder position.

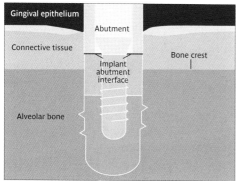

Supracrestal implant shoulder position.
(Redrawn from Broggini et al[25] with permission.)

Implant site   Edentulous area in the alveolar ridge where an implant is planned for support of a restoration.

Implant site development   Alveolar ridge augmentation for future implant placement; requires a staged approach.   See also: *Alveolar ridge augmentation.*

Implant soft tissue management   Procedures performed to maintain periodontal health of the soft tissues surrounding oral implants, including nonsurgical procedures such as scaling, polishing, and oral hygiene instruction at defined intervals.

Implant splinting   Act of connecting dental implants to each other or natural teeth to enhance the strength, stability, and stress distribution of the supporting units.[8]   See: *Splinting.*

Implant stability   Relative mobility of an implant in relation to its surrounding bone when tested manually or with a motion-sensing device.   See also: *Stability.*

Finite element analysis and i. s.
   See: *Finite element analysis (FEA).*

Implant stability quotient (ISQ)   Ratio used to evaluate implant and/or abutment stability using resonance frequency analysis (RFA).   See also: *Resonance frequency analysis (RFA).*

Implant stiffness   Stiffness or rigidity of an implant body as determined by mechanical testing. Influenced by implant body design, composition and diameter.   See also: *Moment of inertia.*

Implant success   See: *Success rate.*

Implant-supported prosthesis (ISP)   Replacement for missing natural teeth that receives retention, support, and stability from dental implants.[6,7]

Finite element model and i. s. p.   Computer-generated models of implant-supported prostheses.   See also: *Finite element analysis (FEA).*

Rigidity of i. s. p.   Relative stiffness of an implant prosthesis. Rigidity is affected by the materials used to fabricate the prosthesis, and the cross sectional area and shape of the prosthesis.   See: *Moment of inertia.*

Implant surface   External surface of an implant body; the façade of an implant, including its macro and micro surface shape and texture. In the manufacture of an implant, various surface treatments may be used, including, but not limited to, polishing, machining, acid-etching, and grit-blasting, to create the desired surface topography.[26,27]   See also: *Acid-etched implant; Anisotropic implant surface;*

Grit-blasted implant surface; Hydroxyapatite implant surface; Rough implant surface; Sand-blasted implant surface; Sandblasted, large-grit, acid-etched (SLA*) implant surface; Sub-tracted implant surface; Turned implant sur-face.

Implant surgery Surgical procedure involving the placement of an implant.

Implant survival Existence of an implant in the oral cavity under stated criteria. It is generally considered desirable to maximize the bone-implant contact (BIC) (ie, osseointegration) of a functionally loaded implant. It can be as-sumed, subjectively, that increased BIC is asso-ciated with high implant survival. See also: *Survival rate.*

Implant system Group of devices or artificial objects combined for use in a common pur-pose. Implant systems include all hardware and related instruments/devices used for their application.[14,28]

Implant thread Varied geometric extrusion from the body of a metal implant. Specific de-sign feature of a threaded implant that is manufacturer specific. There are basics in standard screw thread design related to the geometry of a screw. Variations between manufacturers are based on the pitch or slant of the thread and the frequency or number of threads per millimeter along the length of the anchorage component.[29,30] See also: *Thread-ed implant.*

Implant type Classification according to anatomic position, material composition, configuration, shape, surface, and/or implant-tissue interface. Type of implant falls into the choice of classification system and varies among manufacturers.[31]

Implant uncovering See: *Implant exposure.*

Impression Recording of a negative likeness of an object from which a positive reproduction (ie, cast) can be made.[7,8] See also: *Direct (open tray) impression; Implant-level impres-sion; Master impression; Pick-up impression.*

Impression coping Commercially available or custom-fabricated component connected to an implant for the purpose of impression making in the transferral of implant loca-tion or relationship to other implants with-in the dental arch to a laboratory cast.[32] See: *Retained impression coping; Square im-pression coping; Tapered impression coping.*

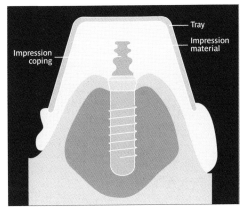

Impression coping (cross section).

I. c. for thread transfer Impression coping used to register the thread timing so as to replicate positioning for the definitive prosthesis.[33]

Impression making Act of recording the neg-ative likeness of anatomic structures in a suit-able medium for a positive reproduction in the form of a cast or moulage. Preferred term to *impression taking.*

Impression taking See: *Impression making.*

Impression tray Container used to transport impression medium to the mouth and to lim-it material flow around the structures to be recorded while the material sets to form an impression.[8]

---

* Trademark by Straumann

Incidence   Rate with which new events or cases occur during a certain period of time.[34] Compare: *Prevalence.*

Incisal   Cutting surface of incisors or canines.[7,8]

Incisal guidance   Effect of anterior maxillary and mandibular contacting teeth on mandibular movements. When an occlusal scheme is developed in semi-adjustable and fully adjustable articulators that simulate mandibular movement, the incisal guide pin and guide table provide this influence, which is under the control of the clinician.[7]

  I. g. angle   Angle formed by the intersection of the occlusal plane and a line formed by connecting the maxillary and mandibular central incisor tips in centric occlusion.

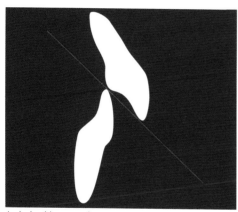

Incisal guidance angle.

  I. g. in semi-adjustable articulator   See: *Articulator, Semi-adjustable; Hanau Quint.*

Incisal guide pin   Adjustable rod attached to one member of an articulator that contacts the guide table on the opposing member to maintain the degree of cast and jaw separation determined in the mouth.[7]   See also: *Articulator.*

Incision   Deliberate cut with a scalpel into gingiva, mucosa, or skin for underlying surgical access.   See also: *Beveled incision; Buccal mucosal incision; Crestal incision; External bevel incision; Internal bevel incision; Releasing incision; Sulcular incision.*

Incision line   Path of an incision through the soft tissues.

Incisive foramen   Foramen of the incisive canal containing the nasopalatal nerve and accompanying blood vessels. It is located just palatal to the two maxillary central incisors along the median suture.

Inclusion criterion   Requirement (such as a diagnostic feature or clinical conditions) that must be met for eligibility to participate in a research project, as specified in the protocol.   Compare: *Exclusion criterion.*

Index   Core or mold used to record and/or register relative positions of teeth, anatomic structures, or implants to one another. The recording medium can have reversible or irreversible characteristics.[7]   See also: *Occlusal index; Remount index; Transfer index.*

Indirect (closed tray) impression   Impression technique by which a stock or custom fabricated tray with impression material is used to record the negative likeness of placed copings. Once the impression material is set and the tray is removed from the mouth, the copings are removed from the mouth and seated in the impression with attached laboratory analogs prior to pouring a cast.[6]

Infection   Localized collection and growth of bacteria that cannot be contained by the host and must be eliminated by systemic antibiotics and/or incision and drainage. Clinically, a distinction is made between acute and chronic infections.   See also: *Acute infection; Chronic infection.*

Inferior alveolar artery [*arteria alveolaris inferior*]   Runs with the inferior alveolar nerve and enters the mandibular foramen at the medial aspect of the ramus. It continues through the mandibular canal with the nerve to the mental foramen, where it divides into the mental and incisive branches.

Inferior alveolar canal   See: *Mandibular canal.*

Inferior alveolar nerve   See: *Alveolar nerve.*

Inflammation   A localized protective response elicited by proximate microbes and/or tissue injury, which serves to destroy, dilute, or wall off both the injurious agent and the injured tissue. It is marked by capillary dilatation, leukocytic infiltration, redness, heat, pain, swelling, and often loss of function.

Acute i.   Intense, localized inflammation, which is the cellular and vascular reaction to injury.

Chronic i.   Inflammation of slow progression that tends to persist long-term (from weeks to years). It occurs when the injuring agent persists in the lesion and the host tissues respond in a manner that is not sufficient to overcome completely the continuing effects of the injuring agent. It may be a continuation of an acute or a prolonged low-grade inflammation and usually causes permanent tissue damage. Chronic inflammation localized to the oral soft tissues, including alveolar and gingival mucosa.

Informed consent   Principle of biomedical research stating that study participants have the right to know the risks and the benefits involved in participating in a research study and that they may not be included in such studies without their explicit written consent.

Infrabony   See: *Intrabony.*

Infracture   Surgical fracturing of a bony structure into a neighboring body cavity with the use of hand instruments, such as in the osteotome technique where the maxillary sinus floor is fractured into the maxillary sinus.   See also: *Osteotome technique.*

Infrastructure   Ceramic or metal implant-supported structure to which a secondary framework or prosthesis is attached.[6]   See also: *Framework.*

Initial stability   See: *Primary stability.*

Injury   See: *Trauma; Wound.*

Innate immunity   Congenital immunity, based on the genetic constitution of the individual.

Insert   See: *Implant placement; Place.*

Insertion torque   Rotational force applied to an object, usually a screw, during placement and/or tightening.

Instability   See: *Primary stability; Secondary stability.*

Install   See: *Implant placement; Place.*

Insulin 1   Polypeptide hormone that regulates carbohydrate metabolism, which is produced in the Islets of Langerhans in the pancreas. Apart from being the primary effector in carbohydrate homeostasis, it influences fat metabolism by changing the liver's ability to release fat stores. Insulin's concentration (more or less, presence or absence) has widespread effects throughout the body.

Insulin-like growth factor (IGF)   Polypeptides structurally similar to insulin. The IGF family consists of two ligands (IGF-I and IGF-II), two cell-surface receptors (IGF-1R and IGF-2R) and several IGF binding proteins. They control growth, differentiation, and the maintenance of differentiated function in numerous tissues. In oral tissues, IGFs are involved in tooth growth and development, in the biology of several periodontal structures, and in various aspects of salivary gland homeostasis.[35]

Interdental bone height   The distance between the bone crest and the contact point between two teeth.

Interdental papilla   See: *Gingival papilla.*

Interdental soft tissue   See: *Gingival papilla.*

Interdental space   See: *Interproximal space.*

Interferon-gamma (IFN-γ)   One of a group of heat-stable soluble basic antiviral glycoproteins of low molecular weight that are produced by T-cells in response to either specific antigen or mitogenic stimulation. It regulates the immune response (eg, by the activation of macrophages and natural killer cells) and is used in a form obtained from recombinant DNA technology in the control of infections and in the treatment of neoplasias.

Interimplant papilla   See: *Gingival papilla.*

Interim prosthesis   See: *Provisional prosthesis.*

Interleukins   Family of potent and multifunctional proteins that serves as a link between inducer and effector cells during immune and inflammatory responses; involved in the recruitment of immune and inflammatory precursor cells. Some interleukins have been implicated in the pathogenesis of periodontal and peri-implantar diseases.

Interleukin-1 (IL-1)   An interleukin produced by macrophages and monocytes that mediates the host inflammatory response in in-

nate immunity. Two principal forms exist, designated IL-1alpha and IL-1beta, with apparently identical biological activity. At low concentrations, IL-1 principally acts to mediate local inflammation, causing mononuclear phagocytes and endothelial cells to synthesize leukocyte-activating chemokines; at high concentrations IL-1 enters the blood stream and acts as an endocrine hormone.

Interleukin-4 (IL-4)   Lymphokine produced by antigen- or mitogen-activated T cells. Its principal role is regulation of IgE- and eosinophil-mediated immune reactions. It stimulates switching of B cells for production of immunoglobulin E (IgE), is a growth and differentiation factor for T cells (particularly helper T cells [Th2], is a growth factor for mast cells, and stimulates the expression of some adhesion molecules on endothelial cells. Formerly called *B lymphocyte stimulatory factor 1.*

Interleukin-6 (IL-6)   Lymphokine produced by antigen- or mitogen-activated T cells, fibroblasts, macrophages, and other cells that induce differentiation and maturation of B cells and growth of myeloma cells. It activates and induces proliferation of T cells and stimulates synthesis of immunoglobulin and plasma proteins such as fibrinogen.

Interleukin-8 (IL-8)   Chemokine produced by monocytes, endothelial cells, and other cells acting as a chemotactic and activator for neutrophils; may play a role in the extravasation of neutrophils in inflammation.

Intermaxillary relationship   See: *Maxillomandibular relationship.*

Internal abutment connection   Connection between an abutment and implant in which the coronal surface of the implant has a core that is threaded or tapered or has a polygonal design.

Internal bevel incision   Reduces the thickness of the mucogingival complex from the sulcular side. Made from a coronal to apical direction, it is usually accomplished for reducing gingival thickness in the posterior segment.

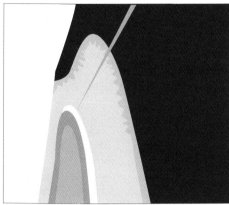

Internal bevel incision.
(Redrawn from Sato[36] with permission.)

Internal distractor   See: *Intraoral distractor.*

Internal hexagon
See: *Hex; Internal abutment connection.*

Internal irrigation   Irrigation of the implant bed through the contra-angle handpiece and drill itself. This irrigation technique has not succeeded in daily practice, since external irrigation seems to be more efficient and cost-effective.   Compare: *External irrigation.*

Internally threaded
See: *Internal abutment connection.*

Interpore   Proprietary product name for porous coralline hydroxyapatite.

Interproximal space   Intervening distance between adjacent teeth in the dental arch.[7,37]

Interpupillary line   Imaginary line connecting the pupils of the eyes. It is useful for evaluating frontal facial symmetry and orientation of the occlusal plane when arranging artificial teeth.[11]

Interquartile range (IQR)   Range of values containing the central half of the observations; ie, the range between the 25th and the 75th percentiles. It is used with the median value to report data that are markedly non-normally distributed.[34]   See also: *Median.*

Interstitial collagenase
See: *Mammalian collagenase.*

Intrabony   Within a bone. Used for description of bony defects or periodontal pockets with their base apical to adjacent bone crest. Called also *infrabony.*

Intramembranous ossification   Bone formation in which connective tissue serving as a membrane becomes a template for bone deposition without any intermediate formation of cartilage. Flat bones are embryonically formed in this way. When sufficient vascularity is present adjacent to the condensed mesenchyme, the osteoblasts begin to produce osteoid. A similar process takes place in healing of bone defects.

Intramobile connector   Implant-abutment connection incorporating a movable or flexible interpositional component intended to modify or reduce the load transferred from the prosthesis to the underlying implant and its surrounding bone. A connector intended to simulate mobility of the periodontal ligament. It was first popularized by Axel Kirsch with the IMZ implant system. Called also *intramobile element.*

Intramobile element (IME)   See: *Intramobile connector.*

Intramucosal insert   See: *Mucosal insert.*

Intraoral distractor   Distraction device designed to be placed within the oral cavity for alveolar distraction osteogenesis. Called also internal distractor.   See also: *Distraction osteogenesis (DO).*

Intraosseous Internal aspect of bone mainly consisting of bone marrow and trabecular bone. Synonym for *endosteal*.

Intraosseous distractor See: *Endosseous distractor.*

Intrasulcular incision Incision approach made along the sulcus of a tooth.

Inverted basket See: *Implant basket.*

Investment casting See: *Lost-wax casting technique.*

In vitro [Latin: *in glass*]. Artificial environment created outside a living organism (eg, a test tube or culture plate) that is used in experimental research to study a disease or process. Compare: *In vivo.*

In vivo [Latin: *in life*]. Biologic processes that take place within a living organism or cell. Compare: *In vitro.*

IQR Abbreviation for *Interquartile range*.

Irradiation Process by which an organ or tissue is exposed to radiation. See also: *Radiation*.

Bone marrow effects and i.
See: *Osteoradionecrosis (ORN).*

Hyperbaric oxygen treatment and i.
See: *Hyperbaric oxygen treatment (HBOT).*

Irrigation Rinsing of the surgical field with a solution. Sterile physiologic saline solution is recommended for this purpose.

Ischemia Blockage or inadequate supply of oxygenated blood to tissues or organs; may be caused by overzealous tight suturing.

Isoforms Approximately 20 BMP family members (isoforms) have been identified and characterized. Each isoform is involved in some developmental process, and BMP-2 has been the most-studied isoform for therapeutic purpose in bone regeneration.[38]

Isograft Tissue graft obtained from a donor who is genetically identical to the recipient.[39]

Isotropic Quality of having the same properties in all dimensions, irrespective of direction.

ISP Abbreviation for *Implant-supported prosthesis.*

ISQ Abbreviation for *Implant stability quotient*.

J

Jig "A device used to maintain mechanically the correct positional relationship between a piece of work and a tool or between components during assembly or alteration."[1]

Joint Articulation of two or more mechanical parts or bones with each other; interface between two or more elements. See also: *Prosthetic joint.*

Joint replacement See: *Prosthetic joint.*

Joint-separating force Tensile force applied to separate two or more contacting components. Generally applied to bolted or friction fit joints.

Junctional epithelium (pl: *junctional epithelia*) Single or multiple layers of nonkeratinizing cells adhering to the tooth or oral implant surface at the base of the gingival sulcus. A long junctional epithelium is an apically extended junctional epithelium resulting from periodontal repair following treatment of periodontal disease. Formerly called *epithelial attachment*. See also: *Epithelium.*

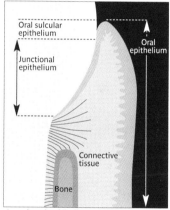

Oral sulcular epithelium
Oral epithelium
Junctional epithelium
Connective tissue
Bone

Junctional epithelium.
(Redrawn from Lindhe et al[2] with permission.)

K

Kaplan-Meier analysis Statistical method used in survival (time-to-event) analysis to estimate the probability of an event, such as implant loss, at different times in the study.[1]

Keratinized gingiva Marginal and attached gingiva that excludes soft tissue of the interdental col region – interproximal gingival tissue between posterior teeth where epithelium is devoid of keratinization.

Knife-edge ridge Severely atrophic edentulous maxillary or mandibular alveolar ridge with a sharp crest resulting from progressive resorption, especially after long periods of denture wearing. "Cawood & Howell class 4 for the anterior maxilla and mandible."[3,4] See also: *Alveolar ridge, Classification of.*

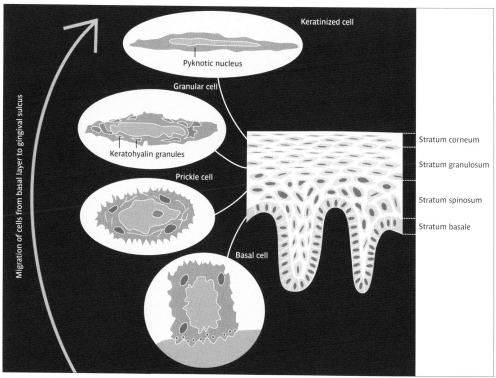

Keratinized gingiva.
(Redrawn from Grant et al[2] with permission.)

L

Laboratory analog Copy of a prosthetic or implant element used in laboratory fabrication procedures.[1] See also: *Analog/analogue.*

Laboratory screw Element used in dental laboratory procedures in the fabrication of the prosthesis. Laboratory screws can be modified, eg, elongated or made from a different alloy, from the definitive design.[2]

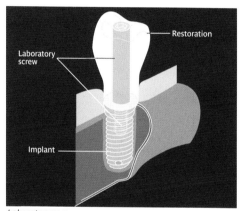

Laboratory screw.
(Redrawn from Yanase and Preston[2] with permission.)

Lamellar bone Adult, mature bone consisting of 3- to 5-µm-wide layers of mineralized collagen fibrils. The orientation of fibrils changes from layer to layer; this construction is often compared with that of plywood. It appears birefringent in polarized light and is found in mature cortical as well as trabecular bone.

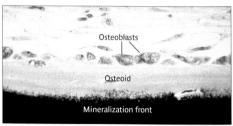

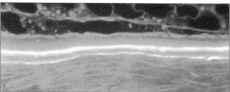

Lamellar bone. (Top: Von Kossatolnidine blue stain; magnification x800. Bottom: Fluorescence after double tetracycline labeling with 1-week-interval-mineralization rate 1 – 2 micron per day.)
(Reprinted from Buser et al[3] with permission.)

Laminate Layered material. In dentistry, a thin layer or veneer of restorative material applied to the surface of a tooth, usually for cosmetic purposes. See also: *Facing; Veneer.*

Lapping tool Instrument used with or without abrasives to improve the adaptation of two opposing surfaces. In the laboratory, an instrument, often rotating, used to remove casting irregularities by means of grinding or polishing.[4]

Laser Acronym for *light amplification by stimulated emission of radiation*; a source that emits photons in a coherent beam that can propagate over long distances without significant divergence and can be focused on very small areas. Can have a very narrow bandwidth, compared with the broad spectrum emitted by most lamps. Light may be emitted continuously or in the form of short or ultrashort pulses, with durations from microseconds to a few femtoseconds. These properties may be the consequence of the very high coherence of laser radiation. Usually includes an optical cavity (resonator), in which light can circulate (eg, between two end mirrors) and which holds a gain medium that serves to amplify the light. See also: *Er:YAG laser; Low-level laser therapy; Nd:YAG laser; Pulsed-mode laser*.

Laser etching Creation of an altered surface by the application of laser energy; frequently used to apply permanent markings to metal objects, such as surgical instruments.

Late implant loss Outcome related to the loss of an implant that occurred after implant osseointegration. Compare: *Early implant loss.*

Late implant placement Implant placement at least 6 months following tooth extraction. The chosen time period should allow for sufficient bone regeneration of the extraction socket, and consequently, implant placement without bone augmentation procedure. Late implant placement bears the risk of bone atrophy in the orofacial direction, particularly in the anterior maxilla.

Latency period See: *Consolidation period.*

Lateral Bennett shift See: *Bennett movement.*

Lateral cephalograph Extraoral radiograph showing the region of the skull that comprises the bones of the face (ie, the viscerocranium). It requires a 18 x 24-cm or 20 x 25-cm image receptor and is intended for diagnosis in orthodontics. It also has been used in the preoperative implant examination to determine size and length of implants to be placed in the interforaminal region.

Lateral window technique Surgical technique using a window into the lateral wall of the maxillary sinus to gain access to the maxillary sinus membrane. Following mobilization and eleva-

tion of the sinus membrane, bone augmentation materials (ie, autografts, allografts, alloplasts, xenografts, or combination mixtures) are used to elevate the sinus floor and allow the placement of dental implants. If the original bone height permits sufficient primary implant stability, then a simultaneous procedure can be used. Otherwise, a staged approach is recommended.[5,6] Compare: *Osteotome technique; See also: Maxillary sinus floor elevation.*

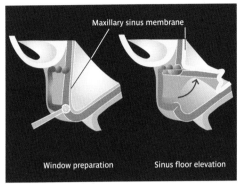

Lateral window technique.

Le Fort I downfracture See: *Alveolar ridge augmentation, Le Fort I downfracture for.*

Le Fort osteotomy Surgical sectioning of the maxilla from the rest of the skull. *Le Fort I osteotomy* sections the midface through the walls of the maxillary sinuses, the lateral nasal walls, and the nasal septum, just superior to the apices of the maxillary teeth. *Le*

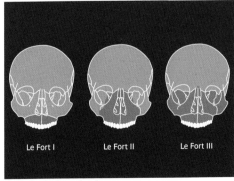

Le Fort osteotomy levels.
(Redrawn from Daskalogiannakis[7] with permission.)

Fort II osteotomy is similar to Le Fort I, except that instead of continuing anteriorly across the pyriform aperture, the osteotomy continues superiorly towards the orbit. *Le Fort III osteotomy* is designed to separate the entire facial mass from the cranial base along the interfrontofacial and interpterygomaxillary planes.[7]

Leukocyte   Blood cell that is colorless, lacks hemoglobin, and contains a nucleus. Leukocytes are involved with host defense and are classified in two large groups: granular leukocytes (basophils, eosinophils, and neutrophils) and nongranular leukocytes (lymphocytes and monocytes). Called also *white blood cell.*

Leukotoxin   Toxin produced by certain bacteria that is specifically destructive to leukocytes, particularly polymorphonuclear leukocytes.

Life table analysis   Study or examination of success/survival rates experienced by a specific population over a particular period of time.[8]

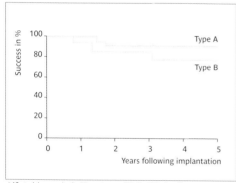

Life table analysis (Courtesy of P. C. O'Brien.)

Lingual   Designation for areas adjacent to the tongue. Often used to identify a tooth surface or ridge segment. Called also *oral.*[9]

Lining cells   Old osteoblasts occupying the surface of mineralized bone with the primary function of nutritional transfer from the surface to osteocytes via cellular extensions. They participate in the normal physiologic re-

modeling of bone by digesting the osteoclast-resistant surface layer, whereby the bone matrix is opened and osteocalcin is released from the bone matrix. The osteocalcin is osteoclast-chemotactic.

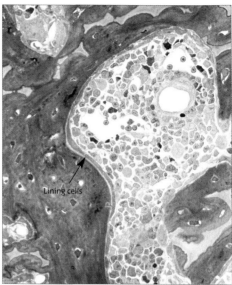

Lining cells (magnification x280). (Reprinted from Garant[10] with permission.)

Lining mucosa
  See: *Alveolar mucosa; Oral mucosa.*

Lip line   Contour of the inferior border of the upper lip at rest or during maximum muscular retraction; reference for position of the residual ridge crest and for orientation of the occlusal plane when planning for esthetics and function during restorative treatment. The *lower lip line* is the relative position of the lower lip at rest or during voluntary retraction.[11]

Lipopolysaccharide (LPS)   A large molecule consisting of lipids and sugars joined by chemical bonds. It is a major component of the cell wall of gram-negative bacteria, a type of endotoxin, and an important group-specific antigen.   See also: *Endotoxin.*

Litigation   See: *Malpractice litigation; Product liability litigation.*

Load   Force applied to an object. In implant dentistry, generally meant to be the placement of a superstructure on an implant to bring it into contact with the opposing teeth during function.   See also: *Occlusal force.*

Loading   Act of applying load to an object. Also, filling a receptacle, such as a syringe.   See also: *Axial loading; Biomechanical load model; Brunski and Hurley model; Delayed loading; Early loading; Immediate loading; Implant loading; Progressive loading; Skalak models of prosthesis loading; Wolff Law.*

   Effects of l. on bone-implant contact   It is generally assumed that loading within a range of physiologic tolerance stimulates increased bone-implant contact, while loading in a magnitude greater than the range of physiologic tolerance may cause loss of bone-implant contact.   See also: *Bone-implant contact (BIC).*

   Effects of l. on framework   Load distribution to supporting implants is affected by the relative stiffness of the prosthesis connecting the implants. With a rigid prosthesis, load is transferred relatively equally to all underlying implants. With a more resilient prosthesis, loading tends to be greatest at the implant closest to the point of load application.[12]

   Screw joint effects on l.   Mechanical effect of loading, usually cyclic in nature, on the stability of bolted or screw-retained joints. Micromotion and fatigue are potential negative occurrences that may result from such loading.

Localized ridge augmentation   See: *Alveolar reconstruction; Alveolar ridge augmentation; Guided bone regeneration (GBR).*

Logistic regression analysis   "Statistical approach to predict or estimate the value of a response variable from the known values of one (termed simple regression) or more (termed multiple regression) explanatory variables. Logistic regression is when the response variable is a binary categorical variable (such as diseased or not diseased) and it can be simple or multiple."[13]

Longitudinal study   Study that follows a patient over an extended period of time.[14]

Lost-wax casting technique   Process of investing a wax or plastic pattern in a refractory mold, then applying heat to melt the pattern, resulting in a void into which molten metal can be cast.[15]

Low-intensity laser   See: *Low-level laser therapy.*

Low-level laser therapy   Type of laser therapy applied for the stimulation of cell function. Unlike high-power surgical lasers used to cut, coagulate, and evaporate tissues for surgical procedures, their biologic effect is not thermal. Called also *bio-stimulating lasers* or *low-intensity lasers.*

LPS   Abbreviation for *Lipopolysaccharide.*

Luting of crowns   See: *Cementation.*

Lymphocyte   Mononuclear, nonphagocytic leukocytes that originate from stem cells and differentiate in lymphoid tissue (as of the thymus or bone marrow). They are the typical cellular elements of lymph and constitute 20% to 30% of the white blood cells of normal human blood. Divided on the basis of ontogeny and function into two classes: B and T lymphocytes, responsible for humeral and cellular immunity, respectively.   See also: *B cell; Macrophage; Mast cell; Monocyte; T cell.*

Lyophilization   Creation of a stable preparation of a biologic substance (eg, blood plasma, serum) by rapid freezing followed by dehydration under high vacuum.   See also: *Freeze-drying.*

M

Machined implant surface
See: *Turned implant surface.*

Macro interlock   Connection between components such as the abutment-to-implant connection that possesses visible (macro) interdigitating or interlocking features.

Macromotion   Motion that is substantial in nature. It is generally applied to the implant body in situations where implant stability is lacking at the time of placement or as a result of loss of osseointegration.

Macrophage   Any of a variety of forms of mononuclear phagocytes in tissues. Derivative hematopoietic stem cell in bone marrow. Relatively large cell with round or indented nucleus, well-developed Golgi apparatus, many endocytotic vacules, lysosomes and phagolysosomes, and a plasma membrane covered with microvilli.

Macrophage-derived angiogenic factor (MDAF)
Macrophage-derived factor that promotes proliferation of new blood vessels. It is released by hypoxic macrophages at the edges or outer surfaces of wounds and initiates revascularization in wound healing.

Magnet   Certain metals or ferromagnetic alloys that demonstrate an attractive or repulsive force between these materials.[1,2]

Magnet attachment system   Retentive mechanism that is nonmechanical but dependent on the attraction properties of rare-earth composition, such as samarium-cobalt and a fer-romagnetic alloy. Elements consist of a magnet and a keeper, which is made of a ferromagnetic alloy.   See also: *Magnetic attachment.*

Magnetic attachment   Retentive device used in removable prostheses requiring the use of a magnet opposing a keeper fabricated of a ferromagnetic alloy.[3]   See also: *Magnet attachment system.*

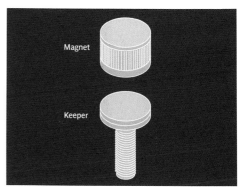

Magnetic attachment.
(Redrawn from Staubli and Bagley[3] with permission.)

Magnetic resonance imaging (MRI)   Imaging that uses magnetic fields and radio waves to produce high-quality two- or three-dimensional images without use of ionizing radiation (x-rays) or radioactive tracers. During an MRI, a large cylindrical magnet creates a magnetic field around the patient through which radio waves are sent. Medical MRI most frequently relies on the relaxation properties of excited hydrogen nuclei in water. The vast quantity of nuclei in a small volume sum to produce a detectable change in a magnetic field, which can be measured from outside the body. When the magnetic field is imposed, each point in space has a unique radiofrequency at which the signal is received and transmitted. Sensors read the frequencies and a computer uses the information to construct an image.

Maintenance   See: *Examination*.

Malpositioned implant   Atypical or faulty position of an implant, rendering it nonusable for restoration. Implant placed incorrectly within the dental arch or prepared site so as to compromise its use.

Malpractice litigation   Legal proceeding in a court or a judicial contest to determine a dereliction from professional duty or a failure to exercise an accepted degree of professional skill or learning by one rendering professional services that results in injury, loss, or damage.[4]

Mammalian collagenase   Proteolytic enzyme that degrades native collagen. After initial cleavage, less-specific proteases will complete the degradation. Collagenases from mammalian cells are metalloenzymes and are collagen-type specific (collagenase 1, collagenase 2, and collagenase 3). They may be released in latent form (proenzyme) into tissues and require activation by other proteases before they will degrade fibrillar matrix. They are involved in the degradation of collagen during tissue repair or during embryonic and fetal development. Called also *interstitial collagenase*.

Mandible   Lower jaw consisting of the horizontal body and two perpendicular rami that end in the coronoid and condylar processes. The condyle articulates in the temporal fossae with the temporomandibular joint.

Cancer-related discontinuity defects of the m.   Defects resulting from mandibular or maxillary tumor resection that require extensive reconstruction. This can be accomplished simultaneously with the resection or in a staged approach. Either vascularized or free grafts are utilized.

Fracture of the m.   Rare complication following implant placement in a severely atrophic mandible or following peri-implant bone loss in an atrophic mandible.[5,6]

Mandibular block graft   Intraoral source of autogenous block graft taken from the patient and fixed to a defect site. The block may be harvested either from the ramus buccal shelf or the mandibular symphysis.

M. b. g. from the ramus   Ramus block graft taken from the buccal shelf area. Advantages include less donor site morbidity; disadvantages include limited block dimension and a low cancellous component.[7]

M. b. g. from the symphysis   Block graft taken from the symphysis region apical to the incisors. Advantages include greater block dimensions, a greater cancellous portion and easier surgical access. Disadvantages include the potential of sensory disturbances following surgery.[8]

Mandibular canal   Bone canal of the mandible in which the inferior alveolar nerve and accompanying vessels are housed.

Mandibular flexure   Deformation of the mandible during function caused by the contraction of the elevator and depressor muscles of the mandible.[9]

Mandibular foramen   Foramen located at the medial aspect of the ramus where the inferior alveolar blood vessels and nerve enter the mandible.

Mandibular movement   Muscle- and ligament-activated border and/or intraborder movements of the lower jaw.[10-12] (See figure next page.)

M

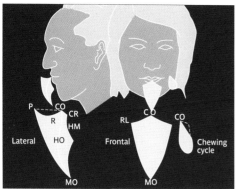

Mandibular movement. P-protrusive; CO-centric occlusion; MO-max. opening; R-rest position; RL-right lateral, CR-centric relation; HM-hinge movement; HO-habitual opening. (Redrawn from Sharry[13] with permission.)

Mandibular overdenture
See: *Implant overdenture.*

Mandibular staple implant
See: *Transosseous implant.*

Marginal gingiva Most coronal portion of gingiva that surrounds the tooth but is not directly attached to the tooth surface. A healthy gingival margin forms the wall of the gingival sulcus. Called also *free gingiva* and *gingival margin*.[14]

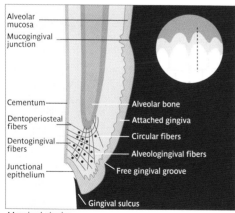

Marginal gingiva.
(Redrawn from Grant et al[15] with permission.)

Marginal peri-implant area That region surrounding the gingival crest adjacent to an oral implant including the interimplant gingival tissue.

Marginal tissue recession
See: *Gingival recession.*

Marrow cavity Central portion of bone between the cortices where marrow is formed.

Mast cell Connective tissue cell with unknown specific physiologic function. Capable of elaborating basophilic, metachromatic, cytoplasmic granules containing heparin, hystamine, and in some species, serotonin.

Master (definitive) cast Final cast used for the fabrication of a prosthesis.[10,16]

Master impression Negative likeness acquired for the fabrication of a cast on which a prosthetic restoration is produced.[10,11,17]

Mastication Act of grinding or crushing food (chewing) preparatory to deglutition and digestion. The masticatory cycle involves three-dimensional movements of the mandible observed in the frontal, horizontal, and sagittal planes.[18] See also: *Mandibular movement.*

Masticatory mucosa Mucosa and gingival tissue that covers the hard palate.

Materia alba Loosely adherent, white curds of matter composed of dead cells, food debris, bacteria, and other components of the dental plaque that lack the organized structure of a biofilm and are found on tooth or oral implant prosthesis surfaces.

Matrix Extracellular substance in which tissue cells (eg, of connective tissue) are embedded. Formative cells or tissue of a fingernail, toenail, or tooth. Mass by which something is enclosed or in which something is embedded (organelles suspended in the cytoplasmic matrix).

Matrix component The part of an attachment that is designed specifically as a receptacle for the matching or mate component (patrix), such that when engaged it provides mechan-

M

ical retention. Attachment systems that use mechanical retention are available in various designs. See also: *Attachment system; Ball attachment system; Bar attachment system; Stud-type attachment system; Telescopic coping attachment system.*

Maxilla Paired bone making up a large part of the facial skeleton, including the body of the maxilla and the frontal, palatine, alveolar, and nasal processes.[19] See also: *Resorbed maxilla.*

> **Computed tomography imaging of the m.** Series of 25 to 45 1-mm axial scans to image the maxilla. For radiation protection, the examined area should be restricted to the region of interest. In implant dentistry, 25 1-mm axial scans have proven sufficient. Effective radiation dose for this examination should range from 2.5 mSv to 6 mSv and, not exceed this value.

Maxillary antrum See: *Maxillary sinus.*

Maxillary artery Artery divided into three parts, based on its location relative to the lateral pterygoid muscle, and further divided into various branches. Different branches supply the mandibular teeth, gingiva, and chin; the maxillary teeth, gingiva, and maxillary sinuses; as well as the hard palate and the lateral nasal walls.[19]

Maxillary cross-arch splint
See: *Cross-arch stabilization.*

Maxillary overdenture
See: *Implant overdenture.*

Maxillary sinus Large pyramidal cavity within the body of the maxilla. Its walls are thin and correspond to the nasal, orbital, anterior, and infratemporal surfaces of the body of the bone. The maxillary sinus communicates with the nose at the infundibulum of the middle meatus through the maxillary sinus ostium.

Maxillary sinus augmentation
See: *Maxillary sinus floor elevation.*

Maxillary sinus floor elevation Augmentation procedure for the placement of implants in the posterior maxilla where pneumatization of the maxillary sinus and/or vertical loss of alveolar bone have occurred. Autografts are often mixed with bone substitutes to increase the volume of the augmentation material or prevent graft resorption during remodeling. Two surgical techniques are well known and routinely used in daily practice: the lateral window technique, first described by Boyne and James in 1980[20]; and the transalveolar osteotome technique, first described by Summers in 1994.[21,22] See also: *Lateral window technique; Osteotome technique.*

Maxillary sinus floor graft Graft used to augment the vertical height in the maxillary sinus for implant placement. A particulate mixture of autogenous bone and a bone substitute is often used. See also: *Maxillary sinus floor elevation.*

Maxillary sinus membrane Thin mucous membrane lining the sinus cavity and characterized by respiratory epithelium. Formerly called *Schneiderian membrane*.

> **Perforation of the m. s. m.** Iatrogenic perforation or tear of the maxillary sinus membrane during sinus floor elevation; the most common complication of this procedure. Small perforations may not need treatment if the elevation can continue uneventfully; larger perforations may be covered by collagen membranes and/or by a fibrin sealant. Incidence of maxillary sinus membrane perforation does not appear to affect the outcome of implant success.[23,24] See also: *Valsalva maneuver.*

Maxillary sinus pneumatization   The maxillary sinuses are usually fluid-filled at birth. Pneumatization, or filling of the sinus cavity with air, takes place during the latter phase of growth as the permanent teeth develop and erupt. Pneumatization can be so extensive as to expose tooth roots with only a thin layer of soft tissue covering them. Later with tooth loss, further pneumatization can take place, leading to a reduced vertical height in the alveolar bone. This often requires sinus floor elevation procedures to allow the placement of dental implants.

Maxillary sinusitis   Infection in the maxillary sinus, either acute or chronic in nature, which can be caused by dental pathology, such as root tips, periapical lesions, overfilled endodontic material, and oroantral fistulae or openings, among others. Acute sinusitis is an absolute contraindication for surgery, whereas, chronic sinusitis is a relative contraindication where implant and/or sinus floor elevation procedures may still be performed.

Maxillary tuberosity   Most distal aspect of the maxillary alveolar process. Bone structure in the tuberosity is often characterized by low density and fatty tissue.[25]

Maxillectomy   Complete surgical removal of the maxilla.

Maxillofacial prosthesis   Restoration replacing oral, stomatognathic, or craniofacial structures with a fixed or removable prosthesis. Support and/or retention is provided by natural teeth and supporting tissues, endosseous implants, or adhesives.[26]

Maxillofacial prosthetics   Branch of prosthetic dentistry concerned with the restoration and/or replacement of stomatognathic and craniofacial structures with fixed or removable prostheses.[11]

Maxillomandibular relationship   Any possible spatial relationship of the mandible to the maxilla.[10,11,27]   See also: *Centric relation.*

  Eccentric m. r.   Any position of the mandible relative to the maxilla other than centric relation or centric occlusion.[11]

McGill Consensus Statement   Conclusion from a 2002 meeting of experts held at McGill University in Montreal, Canada, discussing implant overdenture therapy. Consensus statement on the use of overdentures was that a two-implant supported overdenture was the first choice for restoration of the edentulous mandible and not a conventional denture.[28]

MDAF   Abbreviation for *Macrophage-derived angiogenic factor.*

Mean   Arithmetic average of a group of values. The mean is a common descriptive statistic best used to summarize the central tendency of normally distributed data. In this use, it is usually accompanied by the standard deviation.[29]   See also: *Standard deviation (SD).*

Mechanical failure   Failure of a component caused by mechanical forces. It may be catastrophic in nature or the result of wear, fatigue, or plastic deformation.

Mechanicoreceptor   Nerve ending (receptor) that is excited by mechanical pressure. The mechanical pressure may result from muscle contraction, external pressure (including sound), or touch.

Median   Value that separates the highest 50% of the scores from the lowest 50%. Useful in describing the central tendency of abnormally distributed data, because it is less influenced by the outlier data (ie, extreme values) that skew the distribution and can have a disproportionate effect on the mean.[29]

Medical device Instrument, apparatus, machine, or other related article, including any components (part or accessory), intended for use in the diagnosis of disease or other conditions, for the cure, mitigation, treatment, or prevention of disease in humans.[30]

Medical-grade calcium sulfate A ceramic, the oldest resorbable biomaterial currently in use, which has been used as a filling material in bone cavities for more than 100 years. Calcium sulfate dihydrate [$CaSO_4-2(H_2O)$] (also known as *gypsum*) is mined from the earth.

Medicolegal risk analysis The probability of a patient suffering harm as applicable to medicine and law.

Medullary bone Any substance resembling marrow in structure. Bone formed as an outgrowth from the endosteal lining of the shaft of long bones in birds. The main purpose is accumulation of calcium to be used in the formation of an egg shell. When the shell is being calcified, the medullary bone is destructed and the calcium is released.

Megapascal (MPa) Equivalent to 145 psi (lb/in^2) or 9.87 kg/cm^2.

Membrane See: *Barrier membrane.* See also: *Collagen membrane; Expanded polytetrafluoroethylene (e-PTFE) membrane; Nonresorbable membrane; Resorbable membrane.*

Membranous bone
See: *Intramembranous ossification.*

Mental foramen Foramen from which the mental nerve branch of the inferior alveolar nerve emerges from the mandibular canal; located most often inferior to the apices of the mandibular premolars.[31] See also: *Mandibular foramen.*

Mental nerve The inferior alveolar nerve emerges from the mental foramen as the mental nerve to innervate the skin of the chin and the lower lip.[31]

Mesenchymal cell Type of pluripotential cell that constitutes the mesenchyme.

Mesenchymal progenitor cell (MPC)
See: *Mesenchymal stem cell (MSC).*

Mesenchymal stem cell (MSC) Contributes to the regeneration of mesenchymal tissues (eg, bone, cartilage, muscle, ligament, tendon, adipose, and stroma) and is essential in providing support for the growth and differentiation of primitive hemopoietic cells within the bone marrow microenvironment for the repair of bony defects. The most accessible source of mesenchymal stem cells is bone marrow, although they have been isolated from a number of tissues, including the liver, fetal blood, cord blood, and amniotic fluid.[32] (See figure next page.)

Mesenchyme Mass of tissue that develops primarily from the mesoderm (ie, the middle layer of the trilaminar germ disc) of an embryo. Viscous in consistency, mesenchyme contains collagen bundles and fibroblasts and later differentiates into blood vessels, blood-related organs, and connective tissues.

Mesostructure Intermediate or middle supporting framework connected to the infrastructure and providing support and/or retention for the suprastructure in an implant-supported prosthesis.[17,34]

Meta-analysis Summary and statistical analysis combining the results of two or more studies of similar design to provide a larger sample and more statistical power. It is the statistical technique used in a systematic review to integrate the results of the included studies.[29]

M

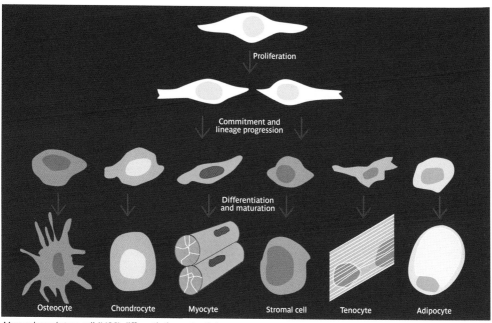

Mesenchymal stem cell (MSC) differentiation potential.
(Redrawn from Goldstein[33] with permission.)

Metal-ceramic restoration Crown or fixed dental prosthesis supported by a natural tooth or implant. It consists of a metal substructure to which a ceramic veneer is fused.[11] See also: *Crown*.

Metal encapsulator See: *Metal housing*.

Metal housing Metallic enclosure in a removable prosthesis into which replaceable plastic retentive elements are placed to stabilize the restoration.[17]

Metal tap See: *Tapping*.

Metaphysis Growing part of a long bone, consisting of the epiphysial cartilage plate united with the diaphysis by columns of trabecular bone.

Methylmethacrylate See: *Resin*.

Metronidazole Antiprotozoal and antibacterial drug ($C_6H_9N_3O_3$) with a spectrum confined to obligate anaerobes, some microaerophilic organisms, and some anaerobic protozoa that act to damage or inhibit DNA synthesis; may induce a disulfiram-like reaction. This antibiotic is commonly used to treat periodontitis and peri-implantitis infections caused by gram-negative anaerobic pathogens.

Microgap Microscopic space between two components, specifically between an implant and an abutment. It is usually considered to be a source of chronic irritation or contamination creating an inflammatory response. See also: *Implant-abutment interface*. (See figure next page.)

M

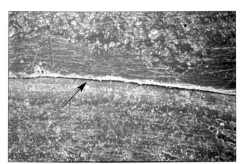

Microgap between implant and machined abutment. (scanning electron micrograph; magnification x200). (Courtesy of T. D. Taylor.)

Microinterlock   Mechanical joining of two or more components through microscopic shapes or undercuts.

Microleakage   Microscopic movement of fluids or contaminants across a barrier or between chambers that cannot be observed without magnification.   See also: *Microgap.*

Micromotion   Relative motion on a microscopic scale. It generally describes the relative motion between an implant and its osteotomy site during the initial healing period or relative motion between mechanical components of the implant stack.

Micromovement   See: *Implant micromovement; Micromotion.*

Microradiography   Radiographic recording of the details within the structure of thin specimens at a high magnification. Also known as x-ray micrography. "The technique of passing x-rays through a thin metal section in contact with a fine-grained photograph to obtain a radiograph which can be viewed at 50 x to l00 x to observe constituents and voids."[35]

Microtextured surface treatment   Treatment providing a microscopically roughened surface.

Microtia   Human developmental anomaly in which there is aplasia or hypoplasia of the pinna of the ear and closure or absence of the external auditory meatus.[10,36]

Midcrestal incision   Incision made on the peak of an edentulous area of the alveolar crest.

Millipore filter   One of the first barrier membranes used as proof of principle for the regeneration of membrane-protected defects. Millipore filters have been used in initial studies for guided tissue regeneration for periodontal defects.[37-41]

Mineralization front   Transitional area of bone mineralization; a seam that separates the osteoid zone from the mineralized part of the bone.   See also: *Tetracycline bone labeling.*

Mini-implant   Implant fabricated of the same biocompatible materials as other implants but of smaller dimensions. Implant can be made as one piece to include an abutment designed for support and/or retention of a provisional or definitive prosthesis.

Minimum effective strain (MES)   Derived from Frost's mechanostat theory for bone adaptation, the MES is essentially a minimum value of strain that must be exceeded to provoke an adaptive response in bone; stimulus for bone remodeling. Called also *minimum effective strain for remodeling (MESr).*[42]

Minimum threshold strain range   See: *Minimum effective strain (MES).*

Misfit   Lack of precise adaptation of one component to another, particularly the lack of ideal passive fit of a multiple-unit prosthesis to two or more implants. Misfit is considered to be detrimental in that it may lead to increased occurrence of component loosening or fracture and may contribute to attachment loss adjacent to an implant.

M

Mobility Presence of relative motion between two objects; eg, the relative stability of an implant in its osteotomy. See also: *Implant mobility.*

Mode Value with the largest number of observations, namely the most frequent value or values.

Model See: *Animal model; Cast.*

Modeling See: *Bone modeling.*

Modified occlusal anatomy Application of nonanatomic occlusal surfaces of artificial teeth in an attempt to control or modify the direction and/or magnitude of forces generated during function or parafunction.

Modulus of elasticity (pl: *moduli of elasticity*) See: *Elastic modulus.*

Moment Rotation of a body when force is applied; the rotary effect of a force.

Moment bending See: *Bending moment.*

Moment of inertia Resistance to rotation of a body; used to explain the relative change if bending moments are based upon the cross-sectional radius of a structure. Called also *I-beam principle* or *second moment principle.* See also: *Implant stiffness.*

Monocyte Mononuclear phagocytic leukocyte, 13 to 25 µm in diameter, with an ovoid or kidney-shaped nucleus. Precursor to a macrophage, it is formed in the bone marrow from a promonocyte and is transported to tissues such as the lung and liver, where it develops into a macrophage.

Morgan and James model of prosthesis loading Model of implant prosthesis loading with rigid implant-to-prosthesis connections.[43]

Morphogen Morphogenetic proteins guiding cellular morphodifferentiation.

Morse taper connection Taper of 3 degrees (6 degrees total convergence) or a reduction of 5/8 inch per linear foot of cylinder length. It describes one method of internal abutment connection, although the Straumann implant-abutment connection to which the term is applied is not technically a Morse taper but rather an 8-degree (16 degrees total convergence) cylindrical taper.

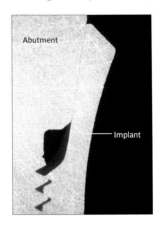

Morse taper connection (scanning electron photomicrograph). (Courtesy of T. D. Taylor.)

Mount See: *Implant mount.*

MPC Abbreviation for *mesenchymal progenitor cell.* See: *Mesenchymal stem cell (MSC).*

MRI Abbreviation for *Magnetic resonance imaging.*

Mucocele "Epithelium-lined sac containing mucus. Mucous cysts in the sinus may appear as spherical, radiopaque areas." Pathologic condition of chronic inflammation in the sinus cavity that is destructive and expansile and can lead to erosion of the sinus walls and possibly life-threatening conditions when in the proximity of the orbit. Radiographically, the presentation is usually a diffuse radiopacity that fills the sinus space and eventually expands beyond the bony walls when erosion of the sinus walls has already taken place. In contrast, a mucous retention cyst represents a benign, usually localized, well-defined opacity at the sinus wall (or within soft tissues, ie, lip). Histologically, a mucocele is lined by respiratory epithelium with extensive goblet-cell metaplasia. Mucous retention cysts are generally asymptomatic, represent a cystic formation of an individual gland and not a contraindication to sinus floor elevation, whereas a true mucocele must first be resolved prior to sinus grafting. Often these two terms are confused with one another.[44,45]

Mucogingival junction   Borderline of union of keratinized gingiva and alveolar mucosa.

Mucogingival surgery   Group of surgical procedures used in periodontics to augment the band of keratinized mucosa around teeth, to cover recession-type defects, or to augment other types of soft tissue defects. Techniques include the use of free gingiva grafts, subepithelial connective tissue grafts, pedicle flaps, use of barrier membranes, among others. Similar techniques have been adopted for implant patients.   See also: *Periodontal surgery*.

Mucogingival therapy   Nonsurgical and surgical treatment procedures for correction of defects in morphology, position, and/or amount of soft tissue and underlying bone support at teeth and implants.[46]

Mucoperiosteal flap   Full-thickness mucosal flap, generally including gingiva, alveolar mucosa, and periosteum. Called also *full-thickness flap*.

Mucoperiosteum   (pl: *mucoperiostea*)   Complex of mucous membrane and periosteum that surrounds and invests the maxilla, mandible, and teeth.[47]

Mucopolysaccharide   See: *Glycosaminoglycan*.

Mucosa   (pl: *mucosae*)   Membrane rich in mucous glands. This is the mucous lining of body passages and cavities that face the lumen, which communicates directly or indirectly with the exterior. It functions in protection, support, nutrient absorption, and secretion of mucus, enzymes, and salts and consists of epithelium, basement membrane, lamina propria mucosae, and lamina muscularis mucosae. Mucosa that covers the dorsum of the tongue is known as specialized oral mucosa. Called also *tunica mucosa* or *mucous membrane*.   See also: *Alveolar mucosa; Masticatory mucosa; Oral mucosa*.

Mucosal button implant   See: *Mucosal insert*.

Mucosal cell   Cells that secrete mucous, such as those found in the oral cavity.   See also: *Mucosa*.

Mucosal insert   Anchorage component placed into soft tissue, an intramucosal anatomic position. "Any metal form attached to the tissue surface of a removable dental prosthesis that mechanically engages undercuts in a surgically prepared mucosal site."[48] Called also *button implant* or *epithelial implant*.

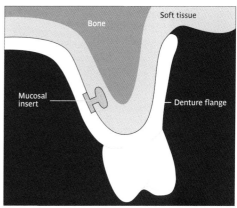

Mucosal insert.

Mucosal peri-implant tissue   Mucosal tissue around dental implants, which forms a tightly adherent band consisting of a dense collagenous lamina propria covered by stratified squamous keratinizing epithelium.[49] The sulcular and junctional epithelium are similar to a natural tooth. The difference is noticed in the connective tissue which is not attached to the implant like in the tooth.[49]

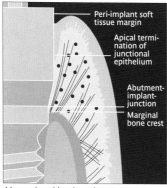

Peri-implant soft tissue margin

Apical termination of junctional epithelium

Abutment-implant-junction

Marginal bone crest

Mucosal peri-implant tissue.
(Redrawn from Misch[50] with permission.)

Mucositis   Inflammation of a mucous membrane, specifically of the mucosal peri-implant tissues.   See also: *Peri-implant mucositis.*

Mucous membrane   See: *Mucosa.*

Multicenter study   Clinical trial carried out at more than one site.

Multidisciplinary treatment   Team approach to provision of patient treatment, encompassing the services of clinicians from various disciplines and adjunct laboratory personnel.[51–53]

Multiple regression   "To predict the value of a single response variable from a combination of explanatory variables."[54]

M

N

N   Abbreviation for *Newton.*

Nasal prosthesis   See: *Nasal reconstruction.*

Nasal reconstruction   Prosthetic restoration of defects of the nose resulting from surgery, trauma, or congenital etiology.[1]

Nasopalatine nerve   One of the terminal branches of the maxillary nerve (second branch of the trigeminal nerve) descending through the hard palate from the incisive canal to supply palatal structures around the central and lateral incisors.[2]

Natural tooth intrusion   Apical movement of a tooth produced by an external force. Phenomenon reported in literature as being a complication of connecting a natural tooth to a dental implant with a fixed prosthesis.[3]

Navigation   See: *Computer-aided navigation.*

Ncm   Abbreviation for *Newton centimeter.*

Nd:YAG laser   Nd:YAG is an acronym for *neodymium-doped yttrium aluminum garnet*, a compound that is used as the lasing medium for certain solid-state lasers. The YAG crystal is doped with triple-ionized neodymium, an active medium that replaces another element of roughly the same size, typically yttrium. Nd:YAG lasers are optically pumped using a flashlamp or laser diodes. One of the most common types of laser, they are used for many different applications. Nd:YAG lasers typically emit light with a wavelength of 1,064 nm, which is in the infrared range. However, there are also transitions near 940, 1,120, 1,320, and 1,440 nm. Nd:YAG lasers operate in both pulsed and continuous mode.

Necrosis   Death of one or more cells or a portion of a tissue or organ; typically characterized by pyknosis (shrunken and darkly basophilic nuclear staining), karyolysis (swollen and pale basophilic nuclear staining), or karyorrhexis (nuclear rupture or fragmentation). It occurs when insufficient blood is supplied to the tissue, whether from injury, radiation, or chemicals. Once necrosis occurs, it is irreversible.   See also: *Osteonecrosis.*

Neoplasm   Abnormal tissue mass that, if malignant, can have the capacity to metastasize locally or systemically. When malignant, the disease entity is generically known as *cancer.*

Nerve lateralization   Surgical procedure that repositions the inferior alveolar nerve for the purpose of implant placement without bone augmentation. The buccal cortex surrounding the mandibular canal is removed to allow the repositioning of the nerve. This procedure raises the risk of neuropathies, such as para-, dys-, and/or anesthesia of the inferior alveolar nerve. Because of the high risk of complications, widespread use has not been achieved.[4-7]

Nerve repositioning   See: *Nerve lateralization.*

Nerve transpositioning
See: *Nerve lateralization.*

Neurovascular bundle Anatomic unit comprising a nerve and its related blood vessels.

Neutrophil See: *Polymorphonuclear leukocyte.*

New attachment Union of connective tissue or epithelium with a root surface that has been deprived of its original attachment apparatus. New attachment may be epithelial adhesion and/or connective tissue adaptation or attachment and may include new cementum.[8]

Newton (N) Unit of force required to accelerate a mass of 1 kg at a rate of 1 m/s²; equivalent to 0.2248 lb or 102 gm.

Newton centimeter (Ncm) Unit of torque. Work performed by a force of 1 N applied at an arm distance of 1 cm.

Newton meter (Nm) Unit of torque. Work performed by the application of 1 N from a distance of 1 m; equal to 1 J.

Nightguard See: *Occlusal guard.*

Nonabsorbable Property of materials that are not capable of being absorbed by the biologic activities of the body.

Nonangled abutment Prosthetic implant component designed to parallel the long axis of the implant; considered straight to indicate no deviation from the long axis of the implant. Called also *nonangulated abutment.*

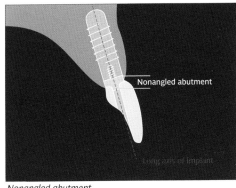

Nonangled abutment.

Nonangulated abutment
See: *Nonangled abutment.*

Nonaxial loading Loading of an implant body that is not along the long axis of an implant body. Compare: *Axial loading.*

Nonbiodegradable Property of tissue substitute that remains unchanged at the site of implantation, with no dispersion in vivo.

Noncollagenous matrix protein Protein presented in the organic matrix of collagen-based calcified tissues together with the supporting collagen meshwork. It contributes to determining the structure and biomechanical properties of the tissues.

Nonfunctional loading Load placed on an implant that is not generated through normal occlusal function or parafunction; for example, applying load through the tightening of an abutment screw.

Nonhexed Property of an implant or a prosthetic component that does not incorporate a mechanical design using a six-sided or six-angled hexagonal elevation or shape.

Nonocclusal loading
See: *Nonfunctional loading.*

Nonresorbable See: *Nonabsorbable.*

Nonresorbable membrane   Membrane made of nonabsorbable biomaterial, most often of expanded polytetrafluoroethylene (e-PTFE). Use of a nonresorbable membrane requires a second surgery to remove it from the site. See also: *Guided tissue regeneration (GTR).*

Nonrotating abutment   Prosthetic implant component designed to prevent rotation of subsequent component, similar to a natural tooth preparation onto which a restoration or other prosthetic component is placed in a predictable position. A portion of the component incorporates a flat side or similar design to prevent 360-degree rotation (ie, spins) of subsequent component.[9-11]

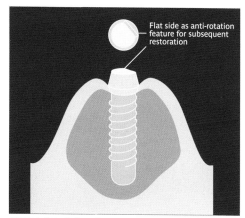

Nonrotating abutment.

Nonrotating gold cylinder   Attachment element designed so that the interface between the gold cylinder and the transmucosal element does not allow 360-degree rotation.

Nonsubmerged healing   Implant placement procedure incorporating a transmucosal extension for healing guidance. Special healing cap is required to extend the implant shoulder above the soft tissue level, allowing the suturing of wound margins around the implant neck/healing cap. This approach does not require a second surgical procedure and is often used in posterior implant sites.[12-13]

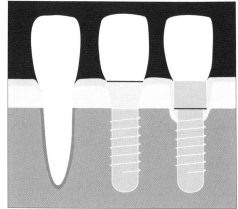

Nonsubmerged healing (center figure).
(Redrawn from Cochran and Mahn[14] with permission.)

Nonsubmerged implant   Implant that is placed with a transmucosal element to allow soft tissue healing immediately after initial placement and to prevent the need for a second surgical procedure. Soft tissue healing occurs around the transmucosal element of either a one- or two-piece implant.   See also: *Nonsubmerged healing; One-piece implant; Two-piece implant.*

Nonthreaded implant   Implant design that does not incorporate threads circumferentially on the external surface of the implant.

Nonvascularized free graft   Graft harvested solely as an osseous graft and without accompanying vasculature.

Nonworking side   Segment of the dental arch (right or left) that is opposite the side at which the teeth occlude during mandibular function.[15]   See also: *Occlusion.*

Normal distribution   Data that have a symmetrical, bell-shaped distribution where the mean, median, and mode are identical.[16]

Null hypothesis   Hypothesis being tested about a population, typically that no difference exists between the mean values of two groups.[16]

N

O

Occlusal adjustment   Modification of the occlusal surfaces of a tooth or teeth to improve form and/or function.

Occlusal anatomy, modified
See: *Modified occlusal anatomy.*

Occlusal force   Force generated by the elevator muscles of the mandible. Occlusal force may be functional (eg, chewing and swallowing) or parafunctional (eg, clenching or bruxing).

Occlusal guard   Removable adjunctive device attached to the incisal and/or occlusal surfaces of the natural teeth or prosthetic restoration for protection from adverse forces related to parafunctional habits, malocclusion, or trauma. It can also be used as a carrier for gels applied to teeth for the treatment of xerostomia and may be fabricated from a resilient or nonresilient material.[1] Called also *bite splint*.

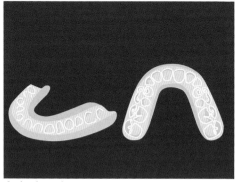

Occlusal guard.

Occlusal index   Record of the intraoral horizontal maxillomandibular relationship. Facial and/or buccal surfaces may also be recorded for repositioning artificial teeth, pontics, or veneers in the laboratory.

Occlusal load   Force applied to natural or prosthetic teeth, implants, and surrounding structures by the elevator muscles of the mandible.   See also: *Occlusal force.*

Occlusal load factor   Force factor involved with occlusal or masticatory function and the resultant loading of underlying teeth, implants or bone.   See also: *Occlusal force.*

Occlusal overload   Application of occlusal loading, through function or parafunction, in excess of what the prosthesis, implant component, or osseointegrated interface is capable of withstanding without structural or biologic damage.

Occlusal table   Collective surface anatomy of the posterior teeth inclusive of molar and premolar cusps, inclined planes, marginal ridges, grooves, and fossae.[2]   See also: *Occlusion.*

Occlusion   The state of being closed or shut off. In dentistry, the occluding of teeth or artificial replacements.[2,3]   See also: *Balanced occlusion; Centric occlusion; Cross-bite occlusion; Disocclusion; Protrusive occlusion; Working occlusion.*

Occlusive membrane   See: *Barrier membrane.*

Ocular implant   Prosthetic conformer placed following enucleation or evisceration of the eye to preserve space for ocular prosthesis.[4]

Ocular prosthesis   Artificial human eye or globe.[4]

Oligodontia   Congenitally related oral condition that presents less than a normal complete natural dentition, often atypically shaped.[3,5]

One-piece abutment   Transmucosal element in which the abutment and attachment mechanism are manufactured as one unit; used instead of a separate fixation screw that threads through the abutment into the implant.

One-piece implant   Anchorage unit and contiguous prosthetic component manufactured as one piece. Implant and transmucosal element as an abutment are manufactured as one component.[6,7]

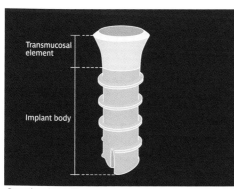

One-piece implant.

One-screw test   Test to determine passive fit when trying in or delivering a multiple-unit implant-supported prosthesis. By inserting a screw in one end of the prosthesis and then observing whether the prosthesis lifts off of other implant or abutment platforms, the clinician can determine the presence or absence of movement when that single screw is tightened, either by clinical or radiographic visualization of the prosthesis relative to the implant-abutment position. Ideally, there should be no movement or lift-off of the prosthesis from its passive seating.

One-stage grafting procedures   Grafting procedures combined with simultaneous implant placement; the remaining bone height must be sufficient for primary stability, and the defect must be self-contained with at least two bone walls.   Compare: *Two-stage grafting procedures.*

One-stage implant   Misnomer for an implant placed with a one-stage procedure.

One-stage implant placement   Protocol that involves one surgical procedure for implant placement. In the single stage the osteotomy site is prepared, the implant is placed, and the transmucosal element exits the soft tissue. Use of a single-stage implant eliminates the need for a second surgical procedure to expose the coronal portion of the implant.

One-stage surgical approach   Category of surgical procedures that can be performed with a single intervention. This group includes standard implant placement with nonsubmerged healing or implant placement with simultaneous bone grafting procedures.

Onlay graft   Graft used in block form and fixed upon the cortical surface of the recipient bed with a screw. Origin may be autograft, allograft, alloplast, or xenograft.

Open curettage   Curettage facilitated by reflection of a soft tissue flap.[8]

Open tray impression
   See: *Direct (open tray) impression.*

OPG   Abbreviation for *Osteoprotegerin.*

Oral   See: *Lingual.*

Oral epithelium   See: *Epithelium.*

Oral health impact profile (OHIP)   Measurement of people's perceptions of the social impact of oral disorders on their well-being.[9]

Oral health – related quality of life   Multidimensional concept assessing how orofacial concerns affect well-being, including functional factors, psychological factors, social factors, and the experience of pain and/or discomfort.[10]

Oral hygiene   Personal maintenance of the cleanliness of teeth and/or oral implants and other oral structures by removal of bacterial plaque and food debris with brushes, dental floss, or other auxiliary devices. Called also *oral physiotherapy* and *plaque control.*

Oral implantology   See: *Implant dentistry.*

Oral mucosa   Mucosa that covers the tissues of the oral cavity.

Oral physiotherapy   See: *Oral hygiene.*

Oral prophylaxis   Removal of plaque, calculus, and stains from exposed and unexposed surfaces of the teeth and/or dental implants by scaling and polishing as a preventive measure for the control of local irritational factors.

Orbital exenteration   See: *Exenteration.*

Orbital prosthesis   Artificial replacement of the contents of the human orbit to contain the globe.   See also: *Ocular prosthesis.*

Orientation index   Mold or form used as a three-dimensional record to register positions between adjacent structures.   See also: *Index.*

Orientation jig   See: *Orientation index.*

O-ring   Retention element resembling a round gasket shape, fitting onto the stud-type patrix of a mechanical attachment. The patrix is soldered or cast to the coping that is cemented into the tooth root.

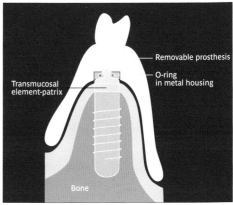

O-ring (cross section).

Oro-antral fistula   Communication created between the sinus and the oral cavity. A true fistula is epithelialized.

Orthodontic anchorage implant   Endosseous dental implant commonly used as anchorage for orthodontic tooth movement. Osseointegrated interface is exceptionally well suited for use as an orthodontic anchor because of its ankylotic nature. Implant may be miniature or standard sized.

Orthodontics   "The area and specialty of dentistry concerned with the supervision, guidance and correction of the growing or mature dentofacial structures, including those conditions that require movement of teeth or correction of malrelationships and malformations of their related structures and the adjustment of relationships between and among teeth and facial bones by the application of forces and/or the stimulation and redirection of functional forces within the craniofacial complex."[5] Called also *dentofacial orthopedics.*   See also: *Immediate loading, Orthodontics.*

O

Orthopantomograph
See: *Panoramic radiograph.*

Orthopedic implant applications Application of osseointegration to orthopedic procedures such as artificial shoulder or hip replacement.

Osseointegration Direct structural and functional connection between ordered, living bone and the surface of a load-carrying titanium implant. (Original definition attributed to P-I Brånemark published in 1985 based on microscopic findings.) The implication is that an interface between an inert metallic surface and living bone is created without an interpositional tissue. Commercially pure titanium (CPTi) and titanium alloy (Ti-6Al-4V) have been proven clinically and microscopically to be biocompatible materials for achieving osseointegration. Osseointegration is considered to be the phenomenon of direct apposition of bone on an implant surface, which subsequently undergoes structural adaptation in response to a mechanical load.[11,12]

Biomechanical failure of o. Loss of osseointegration or failure to osseointegrate initially caused by mechanical forces. During the initial healing phase, comparatively small forces may act to preclude osseointegration from occurring.

Osseoperception Special sensory perception that patients with osseointegrated implants may develop within months following implant placement. A peripheral feedback pathway can be restored, allowing physiologic integration of the implant in the human body and more natural function.[13]

Osseous coagulum Mixture of autogenous bone shavings from areas adjacent to the surgical site mixed with blood. Allogeneic, xenogeneic, or alloplastic graft materials may be added to increase volume and delay resorption.

Osseous coating Bone marrow response to osteophilic surfaces.

Osseous graft See: *Bone graft.*

Osseous regeneration Restoration of original osseous tissue through recapitulation of embryologic events.

Osseous restoration Re-establishment of continuity of osseous tissue; usually restoring form and function.

Osseous rehabilitation Re-establishment of form and function of deficient osseous tissue, aimed at *restitutio ad integrim.*

Osseous repair Restoration of form and function of deficient osseous tissue.

Ossification Formation and development of bone, of which two types are distinguished: endochondral and intramembranous ossification. See also: *Osteogenesis.*

Ostectomy Surgical removal of bone using drills or chisels.

Osteitis deformans See: *Paget disease.*

Osteoblast Mature, polarized, matrix-secreting cell developed from multipotential mesenchymal stem cells via immature and mature osteoprogenitor cells which progress developmentally to preosteoblast and mature osteoblast forms. After a period of function, approximately 10% of osteoblasts turn into osteocytes after stopping matrix extrusion and become entrapped in calcified matrix; the remaining turn into lining cells or undergo apoptosis.

Osteoblast, growth factors secreted by Mononucleated differentiated cells arising from mesenchymal progenitors and associated with the production of bone by secreting bone matrix and enzymes that facilitate mineral deposition within osteoid matrices.

Osteocalcin Protein found in the extracellular matrix of bone, dentin, and the serum of circulating blood. This vitamin K–dependent, calcium-binding protein is produced by osteoblasts and is the most abundant noncollagen protein in bone. Because of calcium-binding sites, it plays a role in bone matrix mineralization or in regulation of crystal growth. In addition, its increased serum concentration is a marker of increased bone turnover in disease states (eg, Paget disease or postmenopausal osteoporosis). It has a low molecular weight and contains three a-carboxyglutamic acid residues per molecule. Called also *gamma-linolenic acid (GLA) protein*.

Osteoclast Cell capable of bone resorption derived from the hematopoietic monocytical cell lineage. Osteoclasts are giant cells with a number of nuclei from 3 to 30 and cell diameters varying from 30 to 100 μm. When actively resorbing, they adhere to the bone surface and produce lacunar grooves called *Howship lacunae*. In the central part of the active osteoclast, the surface is ruffled and hydrogen ions are released for acid production, dissolving the mineral. After mineral dissolution, the exposed fibrils are digested via enzymatic activity.

Osteoclastogenesis Mechanism of osteoclast generation through differentiation of precursor cells of the hematopoietic lineage induced by regulatory molecules. Calcitropic factors, such as vitamin D3, prostaglandin E2, interleukin-1 (IL1), interleukin-2 (IL2), tumor necrosis factor (TNF-alpha), and glucocorticoid induce receptor activator nuclear factor-kappa ligand (RANKL) expression on osteoblasts (see figure). RANKL binding to the RANK expressed on hematopoietic progenitors activates a signal transduction cascade that leads to osteoclast differentiation in the presence of the survival factor colony-stimu-

lating factor 1 (CSF-1). Osteoprotegerin (OPG) produced by osteoblasts acts as a decoy receptor for RANKL and inhibits osteoclastogenesis and osteoclast activation by binding to RANKL.

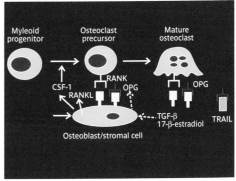

Osteoclastogenesis.
(Redrawn from Theill et al [14] with permission.)

Osteoconduction Physical aid to osteoid formation via species-specific or alloplastic scaffold with nonending porosity.

Osteoconductive graft Autografts, treated allografts, and bone substitutes that provide a scaffold for osteoid formation.

Osteocyte An osteoblast entrapped in the bone matrix during bone formation.

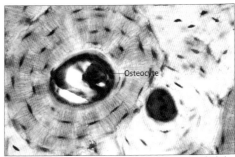

Osteocyte (undecalcified section stained with basic fuchsin; magnification x 250).
(Redrawn from Buser et al [15] with permission.)

Osteodistraction
See: *Distraction osteogenesis (DO)*.

OsteoGen Proprietary product name for an osteoconductive, nonceramic, synthetic hydroxyapatite that is a bioactive, resorbable graft material used for contouring defects of the alveolar ridge. As new bone is formed, it is resorbed over 6 to 8 months. It is composed of a mixture of calcium phosphates.

Osteogenesis Generation, regeneration, and remodeling of bone via concerted action of bone cells. See also: *Compromised osteogenesis; Contact osteogenesis.*

Osteogenetic Quality of any substance, biologic or nonbiologic, that is able to initiate or stimulate normal osteogenesis.

Osteogenic Refers to the stimulation of bone formation produced by modulations of natural biochemical processes such as growth factors and bone autografts, that initiate and maintain and/or support bone formation during a healing response.

Osteogenic protein 1
See: *Bone morphogenetic protein 7 (BMP – 7).*

Osteoid The beginning organic matrix of bone. Initial deposit in bone formation starts with the deposition of osteoid, which is secreted by mature osteoblasts at a speed of 1 to 2 µm per day. When concerned with lamellar bone, a matrix comprised of a scaffold of interwoven collagen fibers (mainly type 1) and noncollagenous proteins are sedimented as osteocalcin and bone sialoprotein – unique for the mineralized tissues – as well as osteonectin, osteopontin, and a number of growth factors. The mean thickness of osteoid in lamellar bone formation is 10 µm; when this thickness is reached, mineralization as sedimentation of crystals of carbonated hydroxyapatite [$Ca10(PO_4)6(OH_2)$] takes place.

Osteoinduction Transformation of osteoprogenitor cells to active osteoblasts via paracrine signals to appropriate receptors. Therefore, bone formation is induced by osteoprogenitor cells in heterotopic sites, mostly via endochondral ossification. Traditionally: the initiation of heterotopic bone formation. Biologically: the initiation of osteogenesis via growth factors.

Osteointegration Ankylotic anchorage of a titanium implant in living bone to achieve a solid bond. Histologically and radiographically described by André Schroeder and colleagues in 1991.[16] See also: *Osseointegration.*

Osteomyelitis Infection of the jaw bone in adults, especially the mandible, as a further development of localized infections such as periapical pathosis, tooth extractions, removal of impacted teeth, or fractures. It is caused by oral bacteria, especially anaerobes as Bacteroides, Porphyromonas, or Prevotella. Early stages of osteomyelitis may be treated by removal of focus and administration of antibiotics. In later stages, surgical treatment (ie, decortication) is necessary.

Osteon Cylindrical structure with a diameter of 150 to 300 µm and a length varying from 2 to 10 µm, composed of concentric lamellae of bone surrounding a Haversian canal with a diameter of 50 µm. In this canal nutritive element, nerves, and connective tissue are present. Between the individual osteons and interstitial lamellae, cementing lines are seen. The longitudinal direction of the osteons is parallel to the axis of the bone. Lamellae are birefringent in polarized light because of changing orientation of the collagen fibers. In the trabecular osteon, the lamellae run parallel to the bone marrow interface.

Osteonecrosis Literally, bone death; however, the term designates the localized necrosis of maxillary and mandibular bone as a side effect of using bisphosphonates in the treatment of myelomatosis and metastatic breast cancer as well as in the prevention of osteoporosis. Osteonecrosis is most often located in the mandible and usually occurs in relation to tooth extraction and dental infections. See also: *Osteoradionecrosis (ORN)*.

Osteonectin Most abundant noncollagenous protein in bone. It may have a role in initiation of mineralization, but the exact role is not known. A number of cells, periodontal fibroblasts, and endothelial cells produce osteonectin.

Osteoplasty Surgical recontouring of bone.

Osteopontin Noncollagenous protein with an arginine-glycine-aspartic acid (RGD) tripeptide sequence having specificity toward cell-surface antigens. It is found in the lamina limitans of the bone surface, possibly playing a role in bone mineralization and attachment of osteoblasts and osteoclasts to bone matrix. It forms a cross-link with fibronectin and is found in cement lines, suggesting a function as biologic matrix-bonding agent.

Osteoporosis Generalized bone disorder characterized by low mineral density and a microarchitectural change of the bone with thinning of the cortical bone and reduction in number and size of the trabeculae in trabecular bone. Diagnosis is made by measuring a fall in bone mineral density (BMD) measured via dual-energy x-ray absorptiometry (DEXA).

Osteoprogenitor cell Relatively undifferentiated cell found on all or nearly all of the free surfaces of bone. Under certain circumstances these cells undergo division and transform into osteoblasts or coalesce, giving rise to osteoclasts.

Osteopromotion Sealing off of a bone defect from the surrounding soft connective tissue by placement of a mechanical barrier (membrane), thereby creating a secluded space into which only cells from the walls of the bone defect can migrate. Expanded polytetrafluoroethylene (e-PTFE) is the best-documented membrane material for promoting bone healing and regeneration by encouraging the biologic or mechanic environment of the healing or regenerating tissues; however, resorbable collagen membranes are equal in value.

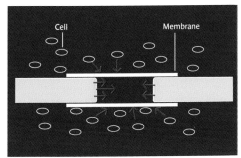

Osteopromotion.
(Redrawn from Buser et al[17] with permission.)

Osteoprotegerin (OPG) Glycoprotein member of the tumor necrosis factor (TNF) receptor superfamily regulating bone resorption by inhibition of osteoclast precursor cells differentiation into mature osteoclasts. It binds to receptor activator nuclear factor-kappa B ligand (RANKL) on osteoblast-stromal cells, thus blocking the receptor activator factor-kappa B (RANK) to RANKL interaction between osteoblast-stromal cells and osteoclast precursors.[18]

Osteoradionecrosis (ORN) Necrosis of jaw bone as a late effect of ionizing radiation, which is used in treatment of malignancies of head and neck. It causes vascular changes with reduction in blood flow resulting in hypovascularity, hypocellularity, and hypoxia. Spontaneous necrosis of jaw bone may appear with subsequent ischemic necrosis of covering mucous membrane and exposure of the necrotic bone to the oral cavity with a secondary invasion of the necrotic bone with microorganisms. Called also *radiation-damaged bone* and *soft tissues*.

Osteotome Circular shafted instrument used to increase dimensions of an osteotomy laterally or apically; available in various dimensions.

O

Osteotome sinus floor elevation
See: *Osteotome technique.*

Osteotome technique Surgical technique using a transalveolar approach to elevate the sinus floor by using osteotome instruments. Anatomic aspects, such as an oblique sinus floor or insufficient bone height, can limit the use of this delicate surgical technique in daily practice.[19,20] Compare: *Lateral window technique.* See also: *Maxillary sinus floor elevation.*

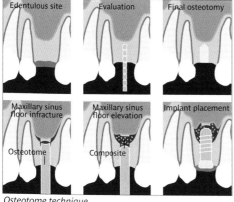

Osteotome technique.

Osteotomy Cut in bone. See also: *Horizontal osteotomy; Pilot osteotomy.*

Ostium of the maxillary sinus Communication between the maxillary sinus and the nasal cavity located at the middle meatus.

Outcome Variable determined prior to experimentation to be the result of the study.

Outcome, primary One outcome determined to be the principal result of an experimental study.

Outcome, secondary Outcome other than the primary outcome of a study that is also of interest in the experimental study.

Overdenture See: *Implant overdenture.*

Overdenture prosthesis
See: *Implant overdenture; Denture.*

Overload Application of force to an object in excess of the force it was intended or designed to withstand. It has the potential for causing permanent deformation or damage to the structure or its support. See also: *Occlusal overload.*

Oxide surfaces Oxygen-containing compounds and complexes formed at the surface of an absorbent. In the case of titanium dental implants, oxidation of the implant surface creates titanium oxide of various chemical formulas through exposure to air or through treatment of the surface at the time of fabrication.[21]

Oxidating surface treatment Creation of metallic oxides on the surface of metal. In the case of titanium, oxidation occurs immediately upon exposure to air. As a result, dental implants made of titanium are coated with titanium oxides critical for the success of osseointegration.

Oxygen therapy See: *Hyperbaric oxygen treatment (HBOT).*

O

P

Paget disease *Osteitis deformans*. Disease of unknown etiology, characterized by enlargement of the cranial bones and often the maxilla and mandible. Cotton-wool appearance of bone on a radiograph may be a diagnostic feature.

Palatal graft See: *Free gingival graft*.

Palatal implant Endosseous implant placed in the hard palate, which is an anatomic location for an implant in the maxilla, or an anatomic location option for use of an implant as anchorage in orthodontic treatment.

Palatal vault Superior surface of the hard palate.

Panoramic radiograph Tomographic survey radiograph of the maxillofacial complex in two dimensions. Image displays the maxilla and the mandible in its curvature and is produced by conventional tomography. Some x-ray machines allow the image to be obtained in sectors.

Papilla (pl: *papillae*) Portion of gingiva extending interdentally below the contact points of two adjacent teeth.

Papilla preservation Measure taken to maintain the interdental papillae following tooth extraction to avoid black triangles between an implant and an adjacent tooth or between adjacent implants. This may include an atraumatic extraction, alveolar ridge preservation, and/or respecting certain parameters when placing implants, such as apicocoronal position and inter-implant distance.

Papilla regeneration Creating a papilla between an implant and an adjacent tooth or between adjacent implants. This may involve surgical procedures using small rotational pedicle flaps, use of connective tissue grafts, and/or prosthetic techniques to condition peri-implant soft tissues. The term is a misnomer, since the papillae flatten in the edentulous space following tooth extraction once the transseptal inserting fibers are lost. A flattened papilla cannot be truly regenerated, but the clinician may optimize its appearance by prosthetic means. The appearance of a papilla is mainly determined by the interdental bone height, which has a documented threshold of approximately 5 mm.[1-4]

Papilla-sparing incision Incision that does not include the papilla and thus avoids the elevation of these tissues.

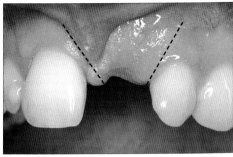

Papilla-sparing incision. (Courtesy of D. Buser).

119

Paracervical saucerization Progressive bone resorption occurring around the cervical portion of implants. Plausible etiologic factors can include: surgical trauma, peri-implantitis, occlusal overload, microgap, implant crest module, and compromise of the biologic width. Also, the excavation of tissue to form a shallow shelving depression, usually to facilitate drainage from infected areas of bone. Called also *craterization*.

Paracrine Transfer of chemical compounds such as hormones and growth factors from cell to cell.

Parallel-fibered bone Repair bone deposited onto woven bone and old bone surfaces in a healing situation as parallel layers of bone. The collagen fibers run parallel to the surface but are not organized in a lamellar fashion.

Parallel(ing) pin See: *Direction indicator*.

Parallel-sided implant Implant with an untapered body when viewed in profile, lengthwise.

Parallel-walled implant
See: *Parallel-sided implant*.

Paresthesia Abnormal sensation of pricking, tingling, or burning related to injury or irritation of a sensory nerve.

Partial denture Fixed or removable dental prosthesis supported and retained by teeth or implants for the replacement of less than a full complement of natural teeth and related hard and soft tissues.[5] Called also *partial prosthesis*.

Implant supported p. d.
See: *Fixed prosthesis*.

Partially edentulous State of being without one or more, but not all, of the natural teeth.[5] See also: *Edentulous*.

Partial-thickness flap Surgical flap that is elevated within connective tissue only, thus leaving the periosteum intact and undisturbed.

Particulate autogenous graft
See: *Autogenous bone graft*.

Particulate graft Graft used in particulate form, which may be an autograft, allograft, alloplast, or xenograft. Particulate grafts differ concerning osteogenic potential, osteoconductivity, hydrophilicity, pore and particle size, and substitution rate.[6-8]

Particulate marrow cancellous bone (PMCB) Graft material obtained from donor sites, such as the iliac crest, with extensive marrow content. PMCB of an autogenous nature is the most osteogenic graft material; the number of multipotential stems cells is especially high.

Passivated surface oxide Surface treatment of an oxidized implant surface resulting in lower surface energy and increased corrosion resistance. This may be the result of intentional treatment of the surface by the manufacturer or simply by exposure to air over time.

Passivation Formation of an oxide layer on the surface of metal exposed to air- and/or oxygen-containing solutions.

Passive fit Adaptation of one component to another in a manner that does not impart strain. In dental implant prosthodontics, the creation of passively fitting prostheses is desirable.

Patient assessment See: *Patient evaluation*.

Patient-based measure Descriptive term referring to the array of questionnaires, interview schedules and other related methods of assessing health, illness, and benefits of healthcare interventions from the patient's perspective. A patient-based outcome measure that addresses constructs such as health-related quality of life, subjective health status, and functional status; used as primary or secondary end-points in clinical trials.[9]

Patient evaluation   Process by which a patient's condition is determined. Called also *patient assessment*.

Patient examination   Clinical examination of the patient, including extraoral and intraoral findings. Called also *control*.   See also: *Examination*.

Patient history   Record of the patient's medical and dental histories.

Patient satisfaction   Individual's perceived fulfillment of a need or a want; can be measured by obtaining reports or ratings from patients about services received from an organization, hospital, physician, or healthcare provider.[10]

Patient selection   Selection of patients who are appropriate candidates for a particular therapy based on risk assessment, including medical, dental, and anatomic factors, as well as smoking habits and psychologic aspects.

Patrix component   The part of an attachment system that is designed specifically to insert and engage the matching receptacle or mate component (matrix) for mechanical retention. Attachment systems that use mechanical retention are available in various designs. See also: *Attachment system; Ball attachment system; Bar attachment system; Stud-type attachment system; Telescopic coping attachment system*.

PDGF   Abbreviation for *Platelet-derived growth factor*.

PDL   Abbreviation for *Periodontal ligament*.

Pedicle flap   Rotated or laterally moved flap receiving its blood supply from the original base of the flap. It is used to cover an adjacent surgical site or improve the thickness of soft tissue contours.[11]   See also: *Soft tissue augmentation*.

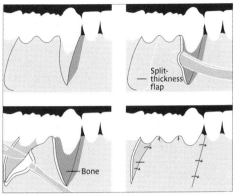

Pedicle flap.
(Redrawn from Ito and Johnson[12] with permission.)

Peer-reviewed journal   Periodical publication for which individuals who are of an academic and/or professional standing equal to that of the author(s) have determined that all articles are of sufficient quality and completeness.

Peer-reviewed literature analysis   Analysis of published research reports by individual(s) with expertise similar to that of the author(s).

Penicillin   A generic name for a related group of natural or semi-synthetic antibiotics derived directly or indirectly from strains of fungi of the genus Penicillium, which exert a bactericidal as well as a bacteriostatic effect on susceptible bacteria by interfering with the final stages of the synthesis of peptidoglycan, a substance in the bacterial cell wall. The penicillins have relatively low toxicity for the host and are active against multiple organisms, especially gram-positive pathogens *(streptococci, staphylococci, pneumococci)*; clostridia; some gram-negative forms *(gonococci, meningococci)*; some spirochetes and fungi. They are classified as penicillin G and congeners (penicillin V), anti-staphylococcal penicillins (methicillin, dicloxacillin), extended spectrum penicillins (ampicillin and amoxicillin), and extended spectrum penicillins with beta-lactamase inhibitors (amoxicillin and clavulanate, ampicillin and sulbactam).[13] See also: *Amoxicillin*.

Percentage bone-implant contact Area of bone in direct contact with the implant surface; usually measured from histologic specimens.[14]

Percutaneous implant Implant placed and positioned through the skin, eg, implants placed extraorally for reconstruction of facial structures or those used in the treatment of fractures in buccomaxillofacial and orthopedic areas.

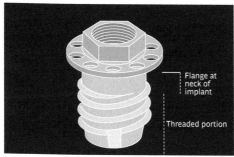

Percutaneous implant.
(Redrawn from Brånemark and Tolman[15] with permission.)

Perforation Inadvertent tear or dehiscence within a flap created during surgery, either by overthinning the mucosa, improper blade direction while making periosteal releasing incisions, or excessive flap retraction.

Peri-abutment Region surrounding an implant abutment. Usually refers to the soft or hard tissues surrounding the abutment.

Periapical radiograph Radiograph taken intraorally showing the entire tooth from the occlusal plane to the apex. The radiograph should reach 3 mm beyond the structures of the tooth.

Pericrestal incision Incision placed not directly over the crest, but in either a more buccal or lingual location.

Peri-implant Around an implant. Often used to describe soft or hard tissues surrounding an oral implant, eg, peri-implant mucosa or bone.

Peri-implant crevicular epithelium Epithelium of the marginal peri-implant mucosa that bounds the peri-implant mucosal crevice and faces the abutment region of the oral implant.

Peri-implant disease Disease that affects the tissues associated with an oral implant and/or abutment. Bacteria play a major role in the etiology of peri-implant diseases, which can be restricted to soft tissue (mucositis) or progress to the supporting bone and induce its destruction (peri-implantitis).

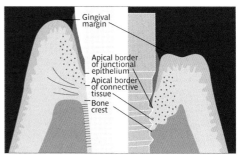

Peri-implant disease (right) compared to periodontal disease (left).
(Redrawn from Grant et al[16] with permission.)

Peri-implant mucositis Progressive bone loss and inflammatory tissue pathology resulting from plaque accumulation and bacterial infiltration around implants.[17]

Peri-implant soft tissue Keratinized or nonkeratinized mucosa around an oral implant.

Peri-implant tissue recession Location of the receding marginal peri-implant tissues apical to the prosthesis-implant interface.

Peri-implantitis   Condition of inflamed peri-implant soft tissues, bone loss, and increased probing depth combined with exudation.

Periodontal abscess   Localized purulent inflammation of the periodontal tissues. Called also *lateral periodontal abscess*.

Periodontal biotype   Categorization determined by variable biologic or physiologic characteristics of periodontal tissue. To evaluate the periodontal biotype, a periodontal probe can be placed at the facial aspect of the periodontal (or peri-implant) sulcus. It is categorized as *thin* if the outline of the underlying probe can be seen through the gingiva or mucosa, or *thick* if the probe cannot be seen.

Thick p. b.   Periodontal biotype characterized by a thick and wide keratinized tissue at the facial aspect of teeth and oral implants. This biotype is prone to pocket formation instead of gingival recession in the presence of periodontal disease.

Thin p. b.   Periodontal biotype characterized by a thin periodontal tissue at the facial aspect of teeth or oral implants. This biotype is prone to gingival recession following mechanical or surgical manipulation.

Thin-scalloped p. b.   Classification of periodontium according to its facial aspects, distinguished by a pronounced disparity between the height of the gingival margin on the direct facial and that found interproximally (ie, noticeable rise and fall of marginal tissue). The underlying bone is usually thin on the facial aspect with dehiscences and fenestrations common.

Periodontal bone regeneration   Regeneration of tooth-supporting alveolar bone that includes new cementum and periodontal ligament (PDL) on the root surface of a previously diseased tooth.

Periodontal disease   General term that includes all pathologic processes that affect the periodontal tissues. They can be restricted to the soft tissues (gingivitis) or involve all the periodontal support tissues (periodontitis) and induce periodontal attachment loss.

Advanced p. d.   Chronic or aggressive periodontitis characterized by clinical attachment loss of 5 mm or more. Teeth with resorption of more than a third of the supporting alveolar bone constitute advanced or severe disease.

Periodontal dressing   Protective material applied over the wound created by periodontal surgical procedures.

Periodontal ligament (PDL)   Specialized fibrous, richly vascular, cellular connective tissue of the periodontium that surrounds the roots of the teeth and is attached to the root cementum, separating it from and attaching it to the alveolar bone. Main functions are to hold a tooth in its socket and to permit tooth mobility and force distribution and absorption by the alveolar process. Called also *periodontal membrane*.

Periodontal maintenance   Procedure performed at selected intervals to assist the periodontal patient in maintaining oral health. As part of periodontal therapy, this procedure is under the supervision of the dentist and not synonymous with a prophylaxis. Called also *supportive periodontal therapy (SPT)*, *preventive maintenance*, and *recall maintenance*.

Periodontal membrane
See: *Periodontal ligament (PDL)*.

Periodontal plastic surgery   Surgical procedure performed to correct or eliminate anatomic, developmental, or traumatic deformities of the gingiva or alveolar mucosa.[18] See: *Mucogingival surgery*.

P

Periodontal pocket Pathologic fissure between a tooth and the crevicular epithelium, limited at its apex by the junctional epithelium; caused by migration of the junctional epithelium along the root as the periodontal ligament (PDL) is detached by a disease process. See also: *Peri-implant disease*.

Periodontal probe Long, thin manual instrument usually blunted at the end and calibrated in millimeters; used to measure the gingival sulcus or pocket depths around a tooth or an oral implant during a periodontal or peri-implant clinical diagnostic examination.

Periodontal regeneration Restoration of lost periodontium, including development of functionally oriented periodontal ligament (PDL), alveolar bone, and gingiva, on the root surface of a previously diseased tooth with de novo formation of cementum.

Periodontal soft tissue Nonmineralized periodontal supporting tissue comprising the gingiva and the periodontal ligament (PDL) tissues; usually refers to the gingival tissues.

Periodontal surgery Surgical procedure for treatment of the periodontium. Includes flap elevation for access, guided tissue regeneration (GTR) for narrow and deep intrabony defects, as well as mucogingival procedures for recession and soft tissue corrections around teeth and implants.

Periodontal treatment Surgical or nonsurgical approaches to the treatment of periodontal diseases.

Periodontitis Inflammation of the periodontal supporting tissues of the teeth from gingiva into the adjacent bone and ligament. Usually a progressively destructive change leading to loss of bone and periodontal ligament (PDL).

Aggressive p. Group of uncommon, often severe, rapidly progressive forms of periodontitis frequently characterized by an early age of clinical manifestation and a distinctive tendency for cases to aggregate in families. Usually there is no contributory medical history, and patients exhibit amounts of microbial deposits inconsistent with the severity of periodontal tissue destruction. Some patients display phagocyte abnormalities and elevated proportions of *Actinobacillus actinomycetemcomitans* and, in some populations, *Porphyromonas gingivalis*. See also: *Periodontal disease*.

Chronic p. Infectious disease resulting in inflammation within the supporting tissues of the teeth and progressive attachment and bone loss; characterized by pocket formation and/or recession of the gingivae. Recognized as the most frequently occurring form of periodontitis, it is prevalent in adults but can occur at any age. Disease is usually associated with the presence of plaque and calculus. Progression of attachment loss usually occurs slowly, but periods of rapid progression can occur. Associated with a variable microbial pattern. See also: *Periodontal disease*.

Periodontium (pl: *periodontia*) Comprises the tissues that invest and support the teeth, including the gingiva, alveolar mucosa, cementum, periodontal ligament (PDL), and alveolar bone.

Periosteal Pertaining to, relating to, or involving the periosteum.

Periosteum (pl: *periostea*) The thin outer surface covering of the mineralized structure of any bone; may be either a delicate connective tissue structure or a dense fibrous membrane (an exception is the articulating surfaces of joints, which are covered by a synovial membrane). Has bone-resorptive and bone-forming

P

potential. Osteoprogenitor cells are located in the vicinity of blood vessels, and the vascular channels in the cortical bone are continuations of the periosteal and endosteal envelope. In adults, it consists of two layers: the external layer being a network of dense connective tissue containing blood vessels and the deep layer comprising more loosely arranged collagenous bundles with spindle-shaped connective tissue cells and a network of thin elastic fibers.

Fibroblastic layer of p.   External of the two layers of periosteum. This network of dense connective tissue contains collagen fibers, fibroblasts, and blood vessels.

Periotest   Instrument used to measure the relative mobility of teeth and dental implants. Device utilizes a tapping piston to percuss a tooth or an implant four times per second. Rate of deceleration recorded at the point of contact is measured as the relative stiffness of the tooth or implant. Periotest values range from -08 to +50, with the -08 to +09 range indicating no discernable movement, +10 to +19 just discernable movement, +20 to +29 obvious movement, and +30 to +50 mobile on pressure.[19]

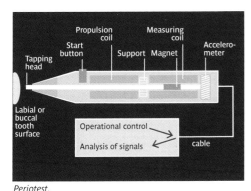

Periotest.
(Redrawn from Falkner et al[19] with permission.)

Periotome   Small pointed or spoon-shaped instrument used to free the ligamentous attachments of a tooth before removal.

Permucosal   Occurring, passed, performed, or effected through the mucosa.

Permucosal extension   See: *Healing abutment.*

Permucosal seal   Seal or tissue barrier at the base of the peri-implant sulcus provided by the epithelial tissue; prevents the penetration of chemical and bacterial substances from the oral cavity to the internal environment of the peri-implant tissues.

PG   Abbreviation for *Proteoglycan.*

PGA   Abbreviation for *Polyglycolic acid.*

Phase-I bone regeneration   First steps in healing of a bone defect with formation of woven bone and consolidation of particulate grafted bone, if used, by bridges of woven bone.

Photon   A quanta that has both wave and particle properties. Has zero invariant mass and travels at the constant speed c, the speed of light in empty space. In the presence of matter, it is slowed or even absorbed, transferring energy proportional to its frequency.

PHSC   Abbreviation for *Pluripotential hematopoietic stem cell.*   See: *Hematopoietic stem cell.*

Physiologic rest position   Passive state of mandibular musculature in which the muscles are in equilibrium in tonic contraction and the condyles are in a neutral, unstrained position. The dentition is nonoccluding.[5,20]

Pick-up impression   Impression of seated superstructure on abutments following surgical implant placement and healing. The superstructure is removed in the impression to obtain a cast incorporating contours of the adjacent soft tissues.[5,20]

Pillar   See: *Stack.*

Pilot drill   Rotary cutting instrument used to create crestal openings in bone for the purpose of directing subsequent osteotomy preparation.[20]

Pilot osteotomy   Initial bone preparation in the series of drilling for implant placement.

PLA   Abbreviation for *Polylactic acid*.

Place   To set in or position an implant in a desired location.   See also: *Implant placement*.

Plaque   Organized mass, consisting mainly of microorganisms, that adheres to teeth, prostheses, and oral surfaces; found in the gingival crevice and periodontal pockets. Other components include an organic, polysaccharide-protein matrix consisting of bacterial by-products such as enzymes, food debris, desquamated cells, and inorganic components such as calcium and phosphate.   See also: *Biofilm*.

Plaque control   See: *Oral hygiene*.

Plasma cell   Antibody-producing B lymphocyte that has reached the end of its differentiation pathway. Plasma cells are oval or round-shaped with extensive rough endoplasmic reticulum, a well-developed Golgi apparatus, and a round nucleus. Principal effector cell involved in humoral immunity. Called also *plasmocyte* or *plasma B cell*.

Plasma B cell   See: *Plasma cell*.

Plasma-containing growth factor   Insulin-like growth factor 1 (IGF-1) is the major growth factor derived from human plasma and found in a variety of tissues and organs including bone matrix.

Plasma spray   Method of attaching material to the surface of a structure such as an implant body. The coating is produced by heating the sintered coating material in an argon environment at extremely high temperatures (>15,000 °C).

The most common plasma spray coatings are titanium and hydroxyapatite plasma sprays.   See also: *Additive surface treatment*.

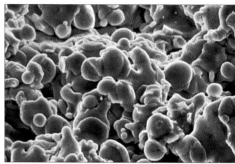

Plasma spray. (scanning electron micrograph; magnification x200).
(Courtesy of D. Buser.)

Plasma-sprayed cylinder   Cylindrical (non-threaded) implant with a surface coating of titanium plasma spray (TPS) or hydroxyapatite plasma spray.

Plasma-sprayed implant   Dental implant with a plasma-sprayed surface.

Plasmid   Extrachromosomal, typically circular double-stranded DNA molecule capable of autonomous replication. Found in the cytoplasm of a variety of bacterial species and often contains genes that confer a selective advantage to the bacterium harboring them (eg, the ability to make the bacterium antibiotic resistant [R plasmid]; conjugation [F plasmid]; produc-

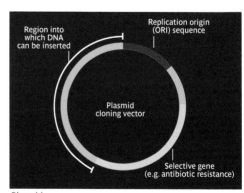

Plasmid.
(Redrawn from Lodish et al[21] with permission.)

tion of enzymes, toxins, and antigens; and the metabolism of sugars and other organic compounds). Plasmids are also used as vectors for gene therapy applications.

Plasmocyte   See: *Plasma cell*.

Plaster   A gypsum material that hardens when mixed with water, used for making impressions and casts.   See: *Dental stone*.

  P. of Paris   Calcium sulfate hemihydrate reduced to a fine powder; the addition of water produces a porous mass that hardens rapidly. It has been used extensively for pouring dental impressions and subsequent casts.

Platelet   Colorless anucleate disk-shaped structure, 2 to 4 μm in diameter, found in the blood of all mammals. It is derived from fragments of megakaryocyte cytoplasm and released from the bone marrow into the blood. Contains active enzymes and mitochondria and has an important role in blood coagulation by adhering to other platelets and to damaged epithelium. Called also *blood platelet*, *thrombocyte*.

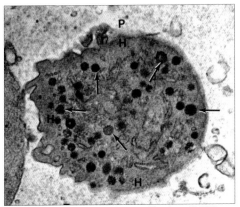

Platelet (electron micrograph; magnification x12,936).
(Reprinted from Berman [22] with permission.)

Platelet-derived growth factor (PDGF)   Mitogenic growth factor found in the granules of platelets and released during blood clotting. It consists of two polypeptide chains linked by bonds containing two sulfur atoms each and regulates cell growth and division (as in connective tissue, smooth muscle, and glia). PDGF plays a role in embryonic development, cell proliferation, cell migration, wound healing, and angiogenesis. PDGF exists in several isoforms based on different polypeptide chains (termed PDGF-A, -B, -C, and -D) and can exist as homo- or heterodimers.

Platelet gel   Platelet concentrate is combined with thrombin and calcium to form a viscous coagulum (gel) used during surgeries to improve adhesive properties and wound-healing characteristics. Additionally, platelet gels form a bioactive matrix that, when activated, releases multiple growth factors that affect tissue regeneration. Platelet concentrate is obtained through a process of differential centrifugation, which can rapidly concentrate autologous platelets and fibrinogen from whole blood. In this process whole blood is centrifuged, and the platelet- and fibrinogen-rich plasma component is harvested.[23]   See also: *Platelet-rich plasma (PRP)*.

Platelet-poor plasma (PPP)   Preparation obtained from whole blood by differential centrifugation. PPP has a relatively high concentration of fibrinogen and is used for autologous fibrin glue preparation, which is employed in surgeries to obtain hemostasis and glue down the flaps.

Platelet-rich plasma (PRP)   Preparation consisting of a limited volume of plasma enriched in platelets and obtained from the patient's blood by differential centrifugation. End product is the platelet fraction, which is suspended in plasma. This platelet concentrate is activated by way of thrombin generation with calcium, resulting in a three-dimensional and biocompatible fibrin scaffold used

P

in regenerative surgical approaches. The autogenous platelets contain a large number of growth factors, including platelet-derived growth factor (PDGF); vascular endothelial growth factor (VEGF); transforming growth factor beta (TGF-β); and proteins, both of which are known to play major roles in soft and hard tissue healing. PRP has been used for a variety of intraoral applications such as maxillary sinus floor augmentation, periodontal or peri-implant bone regeneration as well as a variety of soft tissue reconstructive procedures.[24, 25] See also: *Growth factor.*

Platform   Elevated horizontal surface at the coronal end of an endosseous implant to which components such as abutments or prostheses can be connected.[26]

Platform switching   Act of changing an implant abutment to one with a smaller diameter, so as to place the implant-abutment interface medial to the edge of the implant platform.[26]

Pluripotential hematopoietic stem cell (PHSC)
See: *Hematopoietic stem cell.*

PMCB   Abbreviation for *Particulate marrow cancellous bone.*

PMMA   Abbreviation for *Polymethylmethacrylate.*

Pneumatization
See: *Maxillary sinus pneumatization.*

Polished implant surface   Implant surface intentionally made extremely smooth using abrasives or electrical polishing methods. Compare: *Turned implant surface.*

Polishing cap   An abutment analog or implant analog that is connected to the prosthesis and used to protect the intermediate connection surface during dental laboratory finishing and polishing procedures.[27]

Polyglactin   Type of braided multifilament material made of purified lactides and glycosides. Used as a biomaterial for the synthesis of absorbable sutures and surgical mesh.

Polyglass   Variety of resin-ceramic composite materials for use as direct restorative materials or as computer-aided design/computer-assisted manufacture (CAD/CAM) indirect restorative materials.

Polyglycolic acid (PGA)   Biodegradable, rigid thermoplastic polymer of glycolic acid and the simplest linear, aliphatic polyester used as a material for the synthesis of absorbable sutures and barrier membranes and as a carrier for bone morphogenetic proteins (BMPs). When exposed to physiologic conditions, PGA is degraded by random hydrolysis and apparently also broken down by certain enzymes, especially those with esterase activity. The degradation product, glycolic acid, is nontoxic and can enter the tricarboxylic acid cycle, after which it is excreted as water and carbon dioxide. A part of the glycolic acid is also excreted by urine.   See also: *Guided tissue regeneration (GTR).*

Polylactic acid (PLA)   Biodegradable, hydrophobic, thermoplastic, and aliphatic polyester derived from lactic acid. PLA can be processed in fiber and film and has extensive applicability. In the biomedical field, it is used in a number of applications, including sutures, drug-delivery devices, membranes, and as a carrier for bone morphogenetic proteins (BMPs). Called also *polylactide.*   See also: *Guided tissue regeneration (GTR).*

Polylactide   See: *Polylactic acid (PLA).*

Polymer   Chemical compound or compound mixtures created by molecular reaction to form larger organic molecules containing repeating structural units. A long-chain hydrocarbon.[5,20]   See also: *Resin.*

Polymethylmethacrylate (PMMA) Bone cement, a polymer of methylmethacrylate, which polymerizes in situ with curing temperatures exceeding 100°C; completely nonbiodegradable.

Polymorphonuclear leukocyte Fully developed granular white blood cell whose nucleus contains multiple lobes joined by slender threads of chromatin and cytoplasm; contains fine inconspicuous granules and is stainable by neutral dyes. Comprising up to 70% of the peripheral white blood cells, it is important in infection and injury repair and may have impaired function in some forms of aggressive periodontitis.

Polymorphonuclear neutrophil
See: *Polymorphonuclear leukocyte.*

Polytetrafluoroethylene (PTFE) Homopolymer of tetrafluoroethylene $(CF_2\text{-}CF_2)_n$ that is a nonflammable, tough, inert resin with good resistance to chemicals and heat. Used as a surgical implant material for guided tissue regeneration (GTR), guided bone regeneration (GBR), prostheses such as artificial vessels and orbital floor implants, and for many applications in skeletal augmentation and skeletal fixation. Also used widely in industry, eg, to insulate, protect, or lubricate apparatuses.

Pontic Artificial tooth replacement affixed to a fixed or removable partial prosthesis to restore function and esthetics. Generally locat-

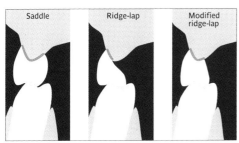

Pontic designs.
(Redrawn from Zarb et al[28] with permission.)

ed in the area of the natural tooth crown(s) being replaced.[5,20]

Porcelain fracture The cohesive failure of porcelain. Etiology of the fracture may be imperfections or stresses residual from fabrication, incompatibility with substrate (thermal coefficient of expansion), substructure deformation because of misfit or inadequate structural integrity, or overload caused by occlusion or trauma.

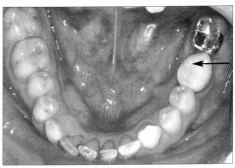

Porcelain fracture. (Courtesy of T. D. Taylor.)

Porcelain-fused-to-metal restoration
See: *Metal-ceramic restoration.*

Porous Property of allowing ingress of fluid or gas within a material or surface; sponge-like quality.

Porous bovine-derived hydroxyapatite
See: *Bovine-derived anorganic bone matrix.*

Porous coralline hydroxyapatite Bone substitute developed from the Porites or Goniopora coral, in which the $CaCO_3$ skeleton of the coral via a hydrothermal process is converted into a hydroxyapatite (HA) substitute with trace levels of β-tricalciumphosphate. It is nonresorbable but osteoconductive because of the nonending porous structure.

Porous marine-derived coralline hydroxyapatite Bone substitute manufactured from calcifying marine algae (*Corallina officinalis*). The process of manufacturing involves pyrolytical segmentation of the native algae and hydrothermal transformation of the calcium carbonate ($CaCO_3$) into fluorohydroxyapatite (FHA [$Ca5(PO_4)3OHxF^{1-x}$]).

Porphyromonas gingivalis Gram-negative, non-motile, anaerobic, non-spore-forming bacillus occurring primarily in the oral cavity and associated with some forms of severe periodontitis. This nonfermentative, pigmented *Porphyromonas* produces a cell-bound, oxygen-sensitive collagenase and is isolated principally from the gingival sulcus.

Posterior dentition Natural teeth or tooth replacements other than the incisors and canines.[20] See also: *Dentition.*

PPP Abbreviation for *Platelet-poor plasma.*

Prefabricated Manufactured in a standardized form or method in anticipation of application.[29]

Prefabricated abutment Prosthetic component manufactured to fit an implant following a design specific to the manufacturer's implant system dimensions.

Preliminary cast Obtained from an initial impression of teeth and associated structures; used for study and/or custom impression tray fabrication.[30]

Preload In bolted joint mechanics, signifies the residual stretch or elongation that remains within the body of the screw after the tightening procedure is completed; the clamping force of the joining screw across a bolted joint.

Premarket notification Submission to the Food and Drug Administration (FDA) for permission to market certain devices intended for human use in the United States of America.[31]

Preparable abutment Prosthetic component that can be modified using rotary instrumentation.

Preparation Planned and executed definitive form of a natural tooth or implant abutment following instrumentation to receive a prosthetic restoration.[20]

Preprosthetic vestibuloplasty Surgical procedure that deepens or lengthens the vestibulum. Several techniques exist, often involving healing by secondary intention or using mucosal or dermal free grafts or split-thickness skin grafts.

Press-fit Joint held together by friction of the parts. Mode of attachment used (either by itself or in conjunction with a screw) by several implant manufacturers for approximating the abutment into the implant body. Also applies to the close adaptation of a root-form (ie, cylindrical) implant to its osteotomy site at the time of placement.

Presurgical consideration See: *Patient selection.*

Prevalence Proportion or rate of persons in a population who had a condition at any given time.[32] Compare: *Incidence.*

Preventive maintenance
See: *Periodontal maintenance.*

Prevotella Intermedium Gram-negative, non-motile, anaerobic, non-spore-forming bacillus isolated from oral and other body sites. A common inhabitant of the gingival crevice, it has been associated with infections of the head, neck, and pleura; also has been associated with inflammatory gingival conditions during pregnancy.

Primary adhesion
See: *Healing by first intention.*

P

Primary bone   See: *Woven bone*.

Primary closure   Surgical wound closure by close flap adaption and complete coverage of the surgical site. This approach leads to healing by primary intention.

Primary implant failure   See: *Early implant loss*.

Primary soft tissue healing
See: *Healing by first intention*.

Primary stability   Clinically, implant immobility at the time of surgical placement, resulting from intimate contact of the implant with the bony walls of the osteotomy. Primary stability decreases with time as osseous remodeling occurs. It is distinct from *secondary implant stability*, which is the result of new bone formation and osseointegration.[33,34]   Compare: *Secondary stability*.

Primary union   See: *Healing by first intention*.

Primitive bone   See: *Woven bone*.

Probing depth   Distance from the soft tissue (gingival or mucosal) margin to the tip of the periodontal probe during usual periodontal or peri-implant diagnostic probing. Measurement can be affected by several factors, such

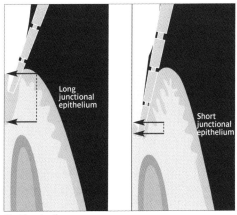

Probing depth.
(Redrawn from Newman et al[35] with permission.)

as the degree of tissue inflammation, the pressure applied on the instrument during probing, the thickness of the probe, and malposition of the probe related to anatomic features.

Product liability litigation   Legal proceeding in a court or a judicial contest to determine if a specific product resulted in injury, loss, or damage.

Profilometer   Instrument used to measure the relative roughness of a particular topography. In dental applications, it is used to measure the relative roughness of implant surfaces.[36]

Progenitor cell   Relatively undifferentiated cells that have the capacity for both replication and differentiation and give rise to one or more types of specialized cells.

   Mesenchymal p. c.   See: *Mesenchymal stem cell (MSC)*.

Progressive loading   Concept of gradually increasing the amount of functional load applied to a newly integrated dental implant or implants by modifying the design and the material of the prosthesis. Based upon the assumption that Wolff Law applies to the bone adjacent to newly osseointegrated dental implants.   See also: *Wolff Law*.

Prophylaxis   Measure taken for the prevention of a disease or condition.   See also: *Antibiotic prophylaxis; Oral prophylaxis*.

Proprioception   Perception of movement and spatial orientation of the body or parts of the body. In the oral cavity, the periodontal ligament (PDL) possesses refined mechanoreceptors that provide highly sensitive neural feedback. This perception is lost or damaged following tooth extraction. It has been proposed that osseoperception of dental implants exists, although on a much lower level than proprioception of natural teeth.[37,38]

P

Prospective study Study planned in advance of data collection. Considered to be more reliable than retrospective studies, because potentially confounding variables can be better controlled when the study question is known before data are collected.[32] Compare: *Retrospective study.*

Prostaglandin Group of lipid compounds derived enzymatically from unsaturated 20-carbon fatty acid, primarily arachidonic acid via the cyclo-oxygenase pathway. They have several hormone-like functions and are potent regulators of a variety of biologic processes, eg, contraction and relaxation of smooth muscle, the dilation and constriction of blood vessels, control of blood pressure, and modulation of inflammation.

Prosthesis (pl: *prostheses*) Artificial replacement for a missing human body part (in dentistry, teeth and adjacent supporting structures and parts of the jaws, face, and cranium). Dental prostheses can replace single, multiple, or all natural teeth and the associated hard and soft tissues.[5,20] See also: *Arm prosthesis; Auricular prosthesis; Craniofacial prosthesis; Definitive prosthesis; Denture prosthesis; Digital prosthesis; Epithesis (prosthesis); Facial prosthesis; Hybrid prosthesis; Immediate restoration; Implant overdenture; Maxillofacial prosthesis; Ocular prosthesis; Partial denture; Provisional prosthesis; Removable prosthesis; Somatoprosthesis.*

Prosthesis bar, Dolder See: *Dolder bar.*

Prosthesis construction Fixed or removable orodental, maxillofacial, or cranial prosthesis. See also: *Restoration.*

Prosthetic joint Artificial replacement for a natural joint. Usually indicated as the result of arthritic degeneration or trauma in a natural human joint.[39]

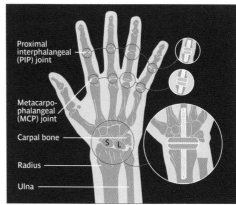

Prosthetic joint. (S = scaphoid; L = unate bone) (Redrawn from Lundborg[39] with permission.)

Prosthetic retaining screw Prosthetic component serving as a retention screw; used to connect the prosthetic component to the mesostructure or to a transmucosal element.[40]

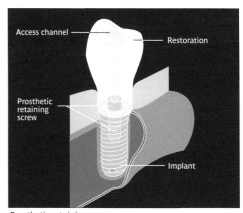

Prosthetic retaining screw. (Redrawn from Yanase and Preston[40] with permission.)

Prosthetic screw
See: *Prosthetic retaining screw.*

Prosthetic table See: *Occlusal table.*

Protein Any of a group of complex organic compounds which contain carbon, hydrogen, oxygen, nitrogen, and usually sulfur, the characteristic element being nitrogen. Proteins, the principal constituents of the protoplasm of all cells, are of high molecular weight and consist essentially of combinations of α-amino acids in peptide linkages. Twenty different amino acids are commonly found in proteins, and each protein has a unique genetically defined amino acid sequence which determines its specific shape and function. Their roles include enzymatic catalysis, transport and storage, coordinated motion, nerve impulse generation and transmission, control of growth and differentiation, immunity, and mechanical support.[41]

Proteoglycan (PG) Extracellular and cell-surface macromolecules derived from a class of glycoproteins of high molecular weight occurring primarily in the matrix of connective tissue and cartilage. Proteoglycans are composed of a protein core with sites for the attachment of one or more polysaccharide chains, particularly glycosaminoglycan; they assemble polysaccharides rather than proteins in their side chains. PGs function in cell adhesion, growth, and organization of the extracellular matrix.

Protocol Precise and detailed set of instructions or directions for performing a study. The instructions state what the study will do and how and why it will be performed. It explains how many subjects will be included, who is eligible to participate (ie, inclusion and exclusion criteria), what and how often study agents or other interventions will be performed, what controls and tests will be included, what information will be gathered, and how the information will be analyzed.[32,42]

Protrusive occlusion Occluding tooth contact when mandibular movement is anterior from centric relation.[5]

Provisional implant Endosseous implant made to smaller dimensional specifications with narrow widths. Can be used for a defined period of time (ie, immediate, temporary, and/or transitional) or to support a transitional prosthesis. See also: *Mini-implant*.

Provisional prosthesis Fixed, removable, or maxillofacial tooth- or implant-supported prosthesis designed and fabricated for limited-term use.

Provisional restoration
See: *Provisional prosthesis.*

Provisionalization Act of planning and fabricating a prosthesis amenable to alteration and use for a limited time period.[43] See also: *Provisional prosthesis*.

PRP Abbreviation for *Platelet-rich plasma*.

Pterygoid implant Implant placement through the maxillary tuberosity and into the pterygoid plate. Treatment approach can be used in patients with severe maxillary atrophy or following tumor resection. Implant is placed into pterygoid bone structure to serve as distal abutments for implant restorations.[44,45] Compare: *Zygomatic implant*.

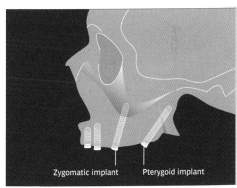

Zygomatic implant   Pterygoid implant

Pterygoid implant.

Pullout force Force applied to dislodge an implant along its long axis and opposite from its direction of placement. See: *Pullout strength.*

Pullout strength Mechanical testing method used to determine the relative resistance to removal of a dental implant. The test may be used immediately following implant placement to determine primary implant stability or at various times following placement and

P

during the healing period. Determines the relative advantages (or disadvantages) of various shapes, materials, and surface textures for dental implants.

Pulsed-mode laser Nd:YAG lasers operate in both pulsed and continuous mode. Pulsed Nd:YAG lasers are typically operated in the so-called Q-switching mode. In this mode, output powers of 20 MW and pulse durations of less than 10 nanoseconds are achieved. See also: *Laser*

Punch technique See: *Tissue punch technique.*

Pure titanium See: *Titanium (Ti).*

***P* value** Probability that an outcome would occur by chance. *P* values (probability values) range from 1 (absolutely certain) to 0 (absolutely impossible). A *P* value equal to or less than 0.05 means that the observed outcome is not likely (≤ 5%) the result of chance.[32]

P

Q

Quality of life   See: *Oral health-related quality of life.*

R

Radiation   Process of emission of energy in the form of waves or particles. When radiation impinges on matter, it is absorbed (ie, transformed), transmitted, or reflected.

Radiation-damaged bone and soft tissues   See: *Osteoradionecrosis (ORN).*

Radiograph   Portrayal of hard tissue structures on film sensitive to x-rays and light.   See also: *Panoramic radiograph.*

Radiographic guide
   See: *Radiographic template.*

Radiographic marker   See: *Radiopaque marker.*

Radiographic prosthesis   Prosthesis that represents the position of missing teeth and dentoalveolar tissues for radiographic imaging. Structure or marking that directs the motion or positioning of something. It is used to transfer the intended position of the implant from the diagnostic cast to the patient and to record its relationship to the underlying bone.   Compare: *Radiographic template; Surgical template.*

Radiographic template   Acrylic resin guide used by the surgeon to direct placement of an implant into its proper position. It is based on the information from two-dimensional panoramic radiographs or three-dimensional computed tomography (CT) or digital volume tomography (DVT) images to achieve optimal implant body placement within the available bone and to preserve vital structures.

Radiology   Medical specialty directing medical imaging technologies for the diagnosis and possible treatment of diseases.

Radionecrosis   Osteonecrosis induced by radiation. It can occur in patients who have undergone radiotherapy because of a malignant process in the ear, nose, and throat (ENT) or other maxillofacial region.

Radiopaque marker   Marker made of metal, or any radiopaque material (eg, radiopaque filling material) that is placed into the mouth before taking radiographs. Detected in the radiograph, the markers help to interpret the image mostly for length, angulation, or localization assessment.

Ramus   Bilateral posterior vertical extensions of the mandibular body. At the superior border, each ramus ends in two processes: the coronoid, which is anterior, and the condyle, which is separated posteriorly by a deep concavity.

Ramus frame implant   One-piece implant of tripodal design consisting of a horizontal supragingival connecting bar with right and left posterior extensions that extend into bilateral ascending rami and one area that extends from the U-shaped frame into the anterior symphysis area. Later design changes incorporated multi-pieces for the same U-shaped frame.[1-3]   (See figure next page.)

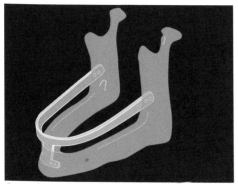

Ramus frame implant.

Ramus graft   See: *Alveolar ridge augmentation; Bone graft, Donor site for; Mandibular block graft, from the ramus.*

Ramus implant   "A type of endosseous blade implant placed into the anterior border of the mandibular ramus."[3]   See also: *Implant type.*

Random assignment   Process of assigning study participants to experimental or control groups at random, such that each participant has an equal probability of being assigned to any given group. This method of assignment helps to prevent bias in a study.[4]

Random controlled trial   Experimental study in which participants are randomly assigned to a treatment or a control group.[4]   See also: *Random assignment.*

Range   Distance between the highest and the lowest values of distribution.

Rank sum test   Comparison of two groups on the median values of the response variable. Called also *Wilcoxon rank sum test.*[4]

RAP   Abbreviation for *Regional acceleration phenomenon.*

Ratchet   Instrument with "a mechanism consisting of a metal wheel operating with a catch that permits motion in only one direction."[5]

RBM   Abbreviation for *Resorbable blast media.*

Reactive bone   See: *Wolff Law.*

Reattachment   To attach again; the reunion of epithelial and connective tissue with root surfaces and bone such as occurs after an incision or injury. It should not be confused with new attachment.[6]

Recall appointment after implantation   Scheduled dental visits after endosseous implants have been placed in a patient.

Recall maintenance
See: *Periodontal maintenance.*

Receptor activator of nuclear factor-kappa B ligand (RANKL)   A 317 – aminoacid peptide, member of the tumor necrosis factor (TNF) superfamily that stimulates osteoclast differentiation and activity as well as inhibits osteoclast apoptosis. It is expressed by osteoblast-stromal cells, fibroblasts, and activated T cells. In the bone tissue, RANKL binds directly to its receptor (ie, receptor activator of nuclear factor-kappa B [RANK]) on the surface of osteoclasts or preosteoclasts, stimulating both the differentiation of osteoclast progenitorcells and the activity of mature osteoclasts. It exists as either a 40- to 45-kd cellular, membrane-bound form or a 31-kd soluble form derived by cleavage of the full-length form at position 140 or 145. It also has a number of effects on immune cells, including activation of c-Jun N-terminal kinase (JNK) in T cells, inhibition of apoptosis of dendritic cells, induction of cluster formation by dendritic cells, and proliferation of cytokine-activated T cells.[7]

Recipient site   Position or site in the alveolar bone crest that is to receive a graft and/or implant.

R

Reconstruction   Restoration of an anatomic organ or structure to its original appearance and function. In dentistry, it is the restoration or replacement of a tooth, teeth, or portion of a jaw or craniofacial structure using an artificial prosthesis.   See also: *Alveolar reconstruction; Prosthesis.*

Record   Information or data recorded in any medium (eg, handwriting, print, tapes, film, microfilm, microfiche, any electronic form). It provides evidence of what was planned, the treatment provided, and the results.

Record base   Temporary prosthesis base used to carry registration materials to the mouth for the recording of maxillomandibular positional relationships.[8,9]   See also: *Maxillomandibular relationship.*

Records, legal requirements for maintaining   Laws that specify the length of time that records must be kept.

Re-entry   Second surgical procedure to place an implant in a staged approach, such as alveolar ridge augmentation or sinus grafting procedures. It can be combined with the removal of an inert biomaterial (eg, nonresorbable membranes or bone graft fixation screws). Can also be performed to improve, enhance, or evaluate results obtained from the initial operation.

Regenerate
See: *Alveolar distraction osteogenesis.*

Regenerate maturation
See: *Consolidation period.*

Regeneration   Regrowth or reconstitution of a lost or damaged body part to restore its former architecture and function.   See also: *Bone regeneration; Guided bone regeneration (GBR); Guided tissue regeneration (GTR); Osseous regeneration.*

Regenerative medicine   Field of medicine concerned with developing and using strategies to repair or replace damaged, diseased, or metabolically deficient organs, tissues, and cells via tissue engineering, cell transplantation, artificial organs, and bioartificial organs and tissues.

Regenerative therapy for alveolar ridge defect   Use of barrier membranes for guided bone regeneration (GBR) to provide a more predictable restoration of form. This method often permits placement of implants simultaneous to defect restoration.

Regional acceleration phenomenon (RAP)   Increase in all metabolic activities in a soft or hard tissue (including modeling and remodeling activity in the skeleton) that is initiated by a provocative stimulus (eg, fracture, crush injury). Typical RAP is induced by periosteal stimulation.[10]

Regression   Class of procedures for predicting the values of a response variable when the value of one or more explanatory variables is known.[4]   See also: *Logistic regression analysis; Multiple regression; Simple regression.*

Rehabilitation   Restoration to a former state of appearance, well-being, and function using artificial replacements.[8]   See also: *Osseous rehabilitation; Restoration.*

Rejection   Immune response to incompatibility in a transplanted organ or grafted tissue that may result in failure of the graft or organ to survive.

Releasing incision   Made to enhance the mobility of a periodontal flap. From the gingival margin or from the base of another incision, it is extended in a vertical or oblique direction.   See also: *Incision.*

Remodeling   See: *Bone remodeling.*

R

139

Remount index   Record of the definitive position of maxillary occlusal surfaces on the articulator for remounting restorations (usually complete dentures) on the articulator for occlusal refinement.   See also: *Index.*

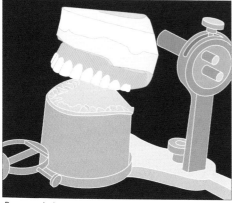

Remount index.

Remount record   Record of positional registration of maxillary occlusal surfaces to be affixed to the lower member of an articulator for occlusal refinement following complete denture prosthesis processing.[9]   See also: *Remount index.*

Removable denture   See: *Removable prosthesis.*

Removable prosthesis   Conventional complete or partial denture or maxillofacial prosthetic restoration readily placed in and removed from the mouth.[9]

Removal torque   Rotational force required to remove an implant from its osteotomy.   See also: *Reverse torque value (RTV).*

Removal torque value
See: *Reverse torque value (RTV).*

Repair   Biologic process where continuity of disrupted or lost tissue is regained by new tissue without restoring structure. Healing occurs via formation of scar tissue. Normal function may not be obtained without restoring structure.

Reparative regeneration   See: *Regeneration.*

Replica   Prosthetic component or element made as a duplicate in every dimension of a specific surgical and/or prosthetic component. A replica can be incorporated in dental laboratory procedures to facilitate making an accurate master cast and/or accurate prosthesis. It can also be incorporated into a model for the purpose of patient education purposes.[11]   See also: *Analog/analogue.*

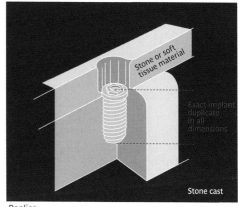

Replica.
(Redrawn from Yanase and Preston[11] with permission.)

Residual abscess   Abscess produced by the residues of a previous inflammatory process, including periodontal or endodontic infection.   Compare: *Chronic abscess.*

Residual ridge   Edentulous part of the maxilla or mandible that once contained the alveolar process. Following removal or loss of teeth, the alveoli heal by new bone formation and remodeling, which leads to some resorptive alterations of the alveolar ridge, especially buccal resorption.[12]   See also: *Alveolar ridge.*

Residual ridge resorption   After tooth removal, alveolar bone undergoes resorption and remodeling. The pattern, timing, and classification for the completely edentulous maxilla and mandible was described by Cawood and Howell in 1988.   See also: *Alveolar ridge, classification of.*

Resin   Organic substance that forms a plastic material following polymerization initiated by heat or chemical activation. It is usually transparent or translucent, not water soluble, and named according to chemical composition, physical structure, or means of activation or curing.[8,13]   See also: *Acrylic resin; Autopolymerizing resin; Composite resin; Epoxy resin; Heat-curing resin.*

Resonance frequency analysis (RFA)   Determination of the relative stiffness of an implant within the bone via attachment of a resonance frequency transducer containing two piezo-ceramic elements to an implant. One piezo element is excited by an electrical signal, and the resulting vibration is measured by the second element. The higher the resulting frequency (in kHz), the stiffer the implant-to-bone connection.[14]

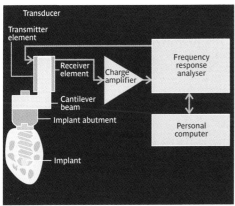

Resonance frequency analysis (RFA).
(Redrawn from Meredith et al[14] with permisson.)

Resorbable   Natural or synthetic material that can be removed by a cellular process, osteoclasts, or foreign body giant cells and macrophages.

Resorbable barrier membrane
See: *Resorbable membrane.*

Resorbable blast media (RBM)   Particles of a resorbable abrasive used to produce a specific surface topography of a dental implant.

Resorbable membrane   Membrane made of absorbable natural or synthetic materials used to avoid a second surgery for its removal. After implantation in the body, membranes are degraded by enzymatic activity (collagen membranes) or by hydrolyses (polylactic acid and copolymers of polylactic and polyglycolic acids membranes).

Resorbed maxilla   Extensive resorption of the alveolar process of the maxilla leads to a nearly complete loss of trabecular bone. Remaining as an alveolar process, it is then almost only a cortical plate, often forming the bottom of the sinus and the nasal cavity.

Resorption   Essential cellular process executed through osteoclastic activity; part of the bone healing process as well as the physiologic remodeling of bone.

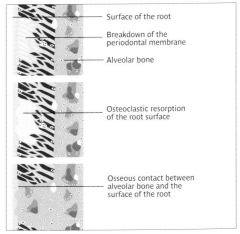

Surface of the root

Breakdown of the periodontal membrane

Alveolar bone

Osteoclastic resorption of the root surface

Osseous contact between alveolar bone and the surface of the root

Resorption.
(Redrawn from Andreasen and Andreasen[15] with permission.)

Resorption quantification
See: *Residual ridge resorption.*

Restitutio ad integrim   Re-establishment of original form and function.

Restoration Material or prosthesis used to restore or replace teeth, parts of jaws, or craniofacial structures.[9] See also: *Acrylic restoration; Osseous restoration; Prosthesis*.

Restorative dentistry Branch of dentistry concerned with the replacement or reconstruction of a tooth or teeth and their supporting structures altered or lost through trauma, surgery, disease, or congenital etiology.[8] See also: *Restorative phase*.

Restorative phase Portion of patient treatment concerned with the diagnosis, treatment planning, and provision of prosthetic therapy.

Restorative platform See: *Platform*.

Retained impression coping Impression coping fixed intraorally either through frictional fit or by being screwed into position. Immediately after removal of the impression, it remains intraorally.[16]

Retainer Device or structure used to retain or stabilize a prosthesis; ie, direct (clasp, clip, or attachment), indirect (partial denture component such as a rest or bar), or restoration (inlay, crown, pontic, among others). In orthodontics, a fixed or removable appliance used to maintain the position and stabilize teeth following treatment.[9,17]

Retaining screw
See: *Prosthetic retaining screw*.

Retention Capacity of a prosthesis or dental restoration to maintain its intended position in function. For a removable prosthesis, the resistance to displacement in the designed path of insertion.[9,18]

Retentive element Portion of a prosthetic component that is the cylinder-to-implant position, directly in contact with the implant.[19]

Retraction cord Slender woven or twisted string-like fabric (usually cotton or similar material) used to retract gingival or mucosal tissues for the exposure of prepared tooth or abutment margins prior to impression making. It is usually impregnated with an appropriate substance to stiffen the cord and provide vasoconstriction.[8,20]

Retractor Instrument used to draw back incised tissues to allow access to a wider operative field or examination.

Retrievability Capacity of a prosthesis, dental restoration, attachment, or screw to be removed without compromising its structure.[21]

Retrospective study Study conducted after data have already been collected.[4] Compare: *Prospective study*.

Reverse articulation See: *Cross-bite occlusion*.

Reverse torque test (RTT) Experimental procedure in which an implant is subjected to unscrewing to determine the relative strength of attachment between the implant and bone. It is usually done on a comparative basis between differing implant surface topographies or roughnesses. It is assumed that the reverse torque value (RTV) will increase as the process of osseointegration progresses. RTT of implants to a torque of 20 Ncm has also been described as a method for determining the success of machined – surfaced, threaded implants in clinical situations.[22]

Reverse torque value (RTV) Resulting value of the torsional force required to unscrew an implant body from its osteotomy. It is assumed that RTV would increase as osseointegration progresses during the healing phase. See also: *Reverse torque test (RTT)*.

R

Revolutions per minute (RPM) Speed at which a shaft turns. It is recorded as the number of complete (360-degree) revolutions the shaft makes in a minute.

RFA Abbreviation for *Resonance frequency analysis.*

Ribbon See: *Articulating tape.*

Ridge See: *Alveolar ridge; Residual ridge.*

Ridge atrophy See: *Residual ridge resorption.*

Ridge augmentation
See: *Alveolar ridge augmentation.*

Ridge defect
See: *Alveolar ridge defect, Implant placement in.*

Ridge expansion See: *Alveolar ridge augmentation, Split-ridge technique for.*

Ridge lap design Tissue-contacting surface of an artificial tooth prepared to accommodate the residual ridge contour on the facial, buccal, and lingual or palatal aspects. A fixed or removable prosthesis incorporating such features may be designated a *ridge lap – designed restoration.*[8,9]

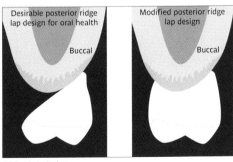

Ridge lap design.
(Redrawn from Stein et al [23] with permission.)

Ridge mapping See: *Bone sounding.*

Ridge preservation See: *Bio-Col technique.*

Ridge resorption
See: *Residual ridge resorption.*

Ridge sounding See: *Bone sounding.*

Ridge splitting See: *Alveolar ridge augmentation, Split-ridge technique for.*

Rigid fixation Process of becoming fixated or rendered immobile, inflexible; applicable to a prosthesis or prosthesis component.[8,21]

Rigidity Stiffness or inflexibility of an object.

Risk assessment Process of predicting an individual's probability of disease.[24]

Risk factor Exposure that has been shown. through data collection and research to increase the probability that a disease or a particular medical condition will occur (eg, smoking is a risk factor for implant failure).[25]

Root "The portion of the tooth apical to the cementoenamel junction that is normally covered by cementum and is attached to the periodontal ligament and hence to the supporting bone."[26]

Root-form implant Inaccurate term often used to describe an endosseous implant. A cylindrical implant does not resemble the root form of a single-rooted natural tooth.[27]

R

Rough implant surface Implant surface with a varying degree of macro- and microirregularity in contrast with a machined or polished, smooth surface. A rough implant surface is generally considered to be superior to a smooth or polished surface in its ability to osseointegrate from both the rate of integration and the relative surface area of bone-implant contact (BIC). Surface roughness of implants can be categorized into three basic levels: minimally rough, 0.5 to 1 µm; moderately rough, 1 to 2 µm; and rough, greater than 2 µm.[28]

RPM Abbreviation for *Revolutions per minute.*

Ruffini receptor Highly sensitive nerve ending of the periodontium in close approximation with collagen fibers that allow refined proprioception around teeth.

Runt-related transcription factor 2 (runx2) See: *Bone morphogenetic protein (BMP); Core-binding factor alpha 1 (CBFα1).*

runx2 Abbreviation for *Runt-related transcription factor 2.*

***R* value** Measurement of roughness of surface topography. Specifically, *R* is the height parameter of roughness, which also includes spacial and hybrid parameters.[29]

R

S

Salivary calculus   See: *Calculus.*

Sandblasted implant surface   Implant surface that has been treated by exposure to silica sand particles propelled under high pressure, thus creating a rough surface texture.   See also: *Rough implant surface.*

Sandblasted, large-grit, acid-etched (SLA*) implant surface   A surface treatment that improves surface roughness to enhance osseointegration through greater bone-implant contact (BIC) as well as an increased rate at which osseointegration occurs.

Sandblasting   Act of modifying or roughening the surface of an implant body by propelling silica sand onto the surface at high velocity under high pressure.

Satisfaction of patient   See: *Patient satisfaction.*

Saucerization   Part of surgical treatment for osteomyelitis in which an essentially closed cavity is opened to the surface by excavation, converting the cavity into a saucer-like defect.

Scaffold   Biocompatible, synthetic or natural supporting structure for growing cells and tissues. It is used in tissue engineering as a carrier of cells or molecules to induce tissue regeneration. In genetics, the chromosome structure consisting entirely of nonhistone proteins remaining after all the DNA and histone proteins have been removed from a chromosome.   See also: *Bone scaffold.*

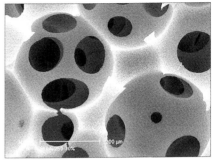

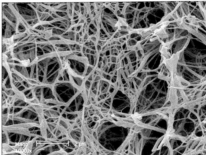

Scaffold (scanning electron micrographs of polymer nanofibrous scaffolds with low magnification at x200 (upper fig.) and high magnification at x100000 (lower fig.)).
(Reprinted from Wei et al[1] with permission.)

Scaffold tissue engineering   Appropriate three-dimensional material with pores and an interconnected pore network with proper surface for attachment, proliferation, and differentiation. It has matching mechanical properties and is bioresorbable with controllable degradation.

S

---
* Trademark by Straumann

Scaler Instrument for removing calculus or other deposits from the surface of teeth or oral implants.

Scaling Instrumentation of the crown and root surfaces of the teeth to remove plaque, calculus, and stains from these surfaces.

Scalloped Curved design of an incision or border, eg, the marginal gingival tissue border.

Scalloped implant A root-form implant design that has the level of the implant-abutment junction elevated interproximally to accommodate the papilla-crestal bone relationship.

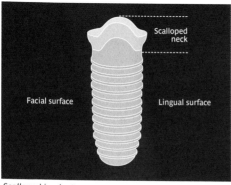

Scalloped implant.

Scanographic template Generic term for a shaped piece of metal, wood, resin, or other material used as a pattern for processes such as painting, cutting out, shaping, or drilling. Examples include a radiopaque marker, radiographic guide, or radiographic prosthesis.

Scar Area of fibrous tissue resulting from the biologic process of wound repair that replaces normal tissues destroyed by injury or disease. Called also *cicatrix*.

Schneiderian membrane
See: *Maxillary sinus membrane.*

Schneiderian membrane perforation
See: *Maxillary sinus membrane, Perforation of.*

Screw "A helically grooved cylinder for fastening two objects together or for adjusting the position of an object resting on one end." The head of the screw has either a groove or slot or other mechanical inset by which it is rotated and driven into something.[2,3] See also: *Abutment, Screw design of; Attachment screw; Closure screw; Coping screw; Cover screw; Prosthetic retaining screw; Sealing screw; Set screw.*

Screw design Common design for cylindrical endosseous dental implants; the screw shape allows for increased primary stability. The time of placement and the screw threads may provide additional load-carrying capacity, although this has not been shown to be significant clinically.

Screw fracture Breakage of occlusal or abutment screws comprising part of an implant supported/retained restoration.

Screw implant
See: *Screw-type implant; Threaded implant.*

Screw joint Interface or junction of two prosthesis components connected by a screw.[4]

Screw loosening Loss of screw preload, resulting in destabilization of a prosthesis or abutment.[4]

Screw preload Clamping or stretching force that occurs across the interface of implant components being attached together via screw tightening. See also: *Preload.*

Screw tap See: *Tapping.*

Screw, Teflon-coated Implant/prosthesis retention screw that has been modified with a polytetrafluoroethylene (PTFE) surface coating.[5] See also: *Screw.*

Screw tightening   Act of turning a screw into its receptacle until resistance is met, resulting in increased tightness of the screw.   See also: *Preload*.

Screw-type implant   An implant with threading on the surface, resembling a screw shape, sometimes referred to as *screw-shape*.   See also: *Threaded implant*.

SD   Abbreviation for *Standard deviation*.

Sealing screw   Healing component used to cover the coronal portion of the implant or as part of a transmucosal healing component that seals the occlusal portion of that component.[6]   See also: *Healing abutment*.

Seating surface   See: *Platform*.

Secondary adhesion
See: *Healing by secondary intention*.

Secondary closure   Misnomer, since the general goal of surgery is to have close flap adaptation and complete closure of the surgical site, and hence healing by primary intention. However, certain situations, incomplete closure is indicated, which leads to healing by secondary intention.   See: *Healing by secondary intention*.

Secondary implant failure
See: *Late implant loss*.

Secondary stability   Implant stability within its prepared bony site, created by osseointegration and the formation of new bone subsequent to loss of the bone initially in contact with the implant at the time of placement. This delayed clinical implant immobility may follow osteotomy site augmentation with bone substitutes and/or healing adjuncts.[7] Compare: *Primary stability*.

Secondary union
See: *Healing by secondary intention*.

Second moment principle
See: *Moment of inertia*.

Second-stage permucosal abutment
See: *Transmucosal abutment*.

Second-stage surgery   See: *Stage-two surgery*.

Seesaw model (of prosthesis loading)   Model describing the mechanical loading aspects of implants or teeth arranged linearly.[8]

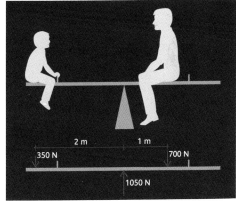

Seesaw model (of prosthesis loading).
(Redrawn from Rangert et al[8] with permission.)

Segmental defect   Resulting defect following removal of jaw segments in tumor patients.

Self-curing resin   See: *Autopolymerizing resin*.

Self-tapping   Ability of certain implant profile designs to cut their own threads into the osteotomy walls at the time of implant placement. A self-tapping implant may be screwed into the osteotomy without first having to pretap the thread grooves.

Semi-adjustable articulator   See: *Articulator*.

Sensory function evaluation   Clinical evaluation that tests sensory function.

Sensory mapping   Anatomic mapping of sensory function that determines if loss or impairment exists. Technique is used longitudi-

S

nally to monitor the improvement of sensory dysfunction.

Septum   Lining or wall separating two cavities or chambers within the body.

> **Maxillary sinus s.**   Cortical bone wall within the maxillary sinus that divides the maxillary sinus floor partially or completely into two or more chambers. Extent of a septum can vary. It is most common in edentulous maxillae, usually located between the second premolar and first molar region, and may cause complications during sinus floor elevation procedures. Called also *Underwood septum*.

Sequestration   Formation of a sequestrum; separation of necrotic bone from the surrounding healthy bone.

Sequestrum   Fragment of nonvital bone that has become separated from the sound, healthy bone during the process of necrosis.

Set screw   Type of retention or attachment screw that is made in smaller dimensions and used to connect a suprastructure and a mesostructure with lingual or palatal horizontal access. Sometimes it is configured as a metal tube with an internally threaded bore and screw system in which prefabricated components are incorporated into the mesostruc-

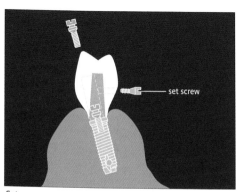

Set screw.
(Redrawn from Staubli and Bagley[9] with permission.)

ture and suprastructures.[9]   See also: *Prosthetic retaining screw*.

Sharpey connective tissue fibers   Terminal portions of principal fibers that insert into the cementum of a tooth. These collagenous fibers pass from the periosteum and are embedded in the outer circumferential and interstitial lamellae of bone. Called also *bone fibers*.

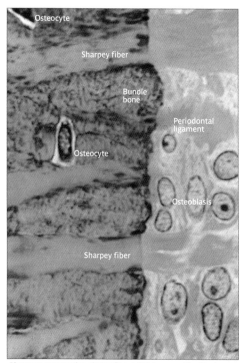

Sharpey connective tissue fibers (high magnification). (Reprinted from Lindhe et al[10] with permission.)

Shear stress   State of stress occurring when two objects in contact are loaded parallel to their surfaces.

Sialoprotein   Noncollagenous protein with a molecular weight of approximately 33,000 KDa that contains the arginine-glycine-aspartic acid (RGD) tripeptide sequence, characteristic for attachment proteins, which interact with cell surface integrins. It has a high calcium-binding potential and binds tightly to hydroxyapatite (HA) as well as to cells.

S

Signaling molecule Molecules that participate in intracellular and intercellular mechanisms involved in chemical transmitting of information between cells. Such molecules are released from the cell sending the signal, cross over the gap between cells, and interact with receptors in another cell, triggering an intracellular signaling cascade that results in a cellular response to the impulse.

Signed rank test Nonparametric form of the paired *t* test for comparing two samples.[11]

Silicone Polymeric organic silicon compound in which some or all of the radical positions that could be occupied by carbon atoms are occupied by silicon. Used for heat- or water-resistant lubricants, binders, and insulators.[12,13]

Simple regression "To predict the value of a single response variable from a given value of a single explanatory variable."[14]

Simulation Imitative representation of the functioning of one system or process by means of the functioning of another. For example, in radiology it could be an image obtained with the same source-to-skin distance, field size, and orientation as the diagnostic beam for visualization of a treated area on a radiograph.[15,16]

Simultaneous implant placement Implant placement with a simultaneous bone-grafting procedure. See also: *Alveolar ridge defect, Implant placement in.*

Single-stage implant Misnomer used for an implant that is placed with a one-stage procedure. See also: *One-stage implant placement.*

Single-stage surgery Used to describe surgical procedures that could be performed in one surgical step. Currently, procedures are described either as a *staged* or a *simultaneous* approach. See also: *One-stage implant placement; Simultaneous implant placement; Two-stage implant placement.*

Single-tooth implant Implant and implant restoration used in a single-tooth gap for the replacement of one tooth.

Sinter Process of fusing small particles or powder into a solid mass through heating.

Sinus augmentation See: *Maxillary sinus floor elevation; Maxillary sinus floor graft.*

Sinus disease Pathology of the maxillary sinus.

Sinus elevation Misnomer used to describe surgical techniques for maxillary sinus floor elevation. See: *Maxillary sinus floor elevation.*

Sinus graft See: *Maxillary sinus floor elevation; Maxillary sinus floor graft.*

Sinus Graft Consensus Conference Conference in which a panel of experts developed and voted on multiple consensus statements derived by committee review of retrospective information for bone–grafting materials, type of implants, timing for implant placement, failure analysis, radiographic analysis, indications and contraindications, prosthetics, and nomenclature. Several consensus statements were obtained, the most significant being that the sinus graft should now be considered a highly predictable and effective therapeutic modality.[17]

Sinus grafting See: *Maxillary sinus floor elevation; Maxillary sinus floor graft.*

Sinus grafting technique See: *Lateral window technique; Maxillary sinus floor elevation; Maxillary sinus floor graft; Osteotome technique.*

Sinus lift Misnomer used to describe surgical techniques for maxillary sinus floor elevation. See: *Maxillary sinus floor elevation.*

Sinus lift surgery Misnomer used to describe surgical techniques for maxillary sinus floor elevation. See: *Maxillary sinus floor elevation.*

Sinus lining
See: *Maxillary sinus membrane.*

Sinus membrane
See: *Maxillary sinus membrane.*

Sinus perforation Oro-antral fistula following tooth extraction or perforation of the maxillary sinus membrane during a sinus grafting procedure.

Sinus pneumatization
See: *Maxillary sinus pneumatization.*

Sinus septum See: *Septum.*

Sinusitis Inflammation of the maxillary sinus from bacterial, viral, fungal, allergic, or autoimmune origin. While acute sinusitis is usually caused by infection with a single type of bacteria or virus, chronic sinusitis is usually caused either by allergies or by infection with several types of bacterium. Infections may be of either dental or otolaryngeal origin.

Site development
See: *Implant site development.*

Site preservation See: *Bio-Col technique.*

Skalak models of prosthesis loading Biomechanical models created by Richard Skalak explaining implant loading by forces applied to an attached rigid prosthesis.[18] (See figure.)

Skin Two-layered outer integument or covering of the body, consisting of the dermis and the epidermis and resting upon the subcutaneous tissues. The outer ectodermal epidermis is more or less cornified and penetrated by the openings of sweat and sebaceous glands, and the inner mesodermal dermis is composed largely of connective tissue and richly supplied with blood vessels and nerves. Called also *cutis.*

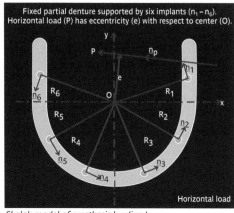

Fixed partial denture supported by six implants ($n_1 – n_6$). Horizontal load (P) has eccentricity (e) with respect to center (O).

Horizontal load

Skalak model of prosthesis loading I.

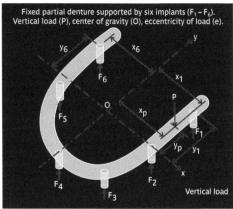

Fixed partial denture supported by six implants ($F_1 – F_6$). Vertical load (P), center of gravity (O), eccentricity of load (e).

Vertical load

Skalak model of prosthesis loading II.

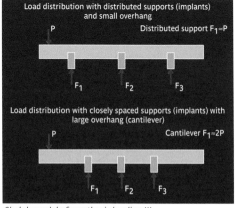

Load distribution with distributed supports (implants) and small overhang

Distributed support $F_1 \approx P$

Load distribution with closely spaced supports (implants) with large overhang (cantilever)

Cantilever $F_1 \approx 2P$

Skalak model of prosthesis loading III.
(Redrawn from Skalak[19] with permission.)

S

Skin-penetrating implant Endosseous implant placed in an extraoral site requiring skin penetration for prosthesis attachment as opposed to wet-surfaced gingiva or mucosa. Maintenance of adequate hygiene in the skin-penetration area can be problematic.[20] See also: *Percutaneous implant*.

Skull simulator Dummy of a skull to elucidate anatomy and execute phantom surgery.

SLA* Abbreviation for *Sandblasted, large-grit, acid-etched*.

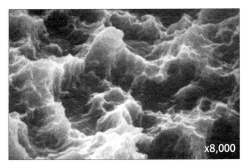

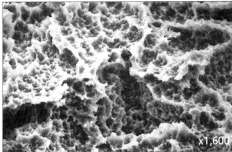

Sandblasted, large-grit, acid-etched (SLA*) implant surface (scanning electron micrograph).
(Reprinted from Cochran et al[31] with permission.)

Sleeper implant Nonfunctioning endosseous implant retained in bone and covered by mucosa for subsequent exposure and/or use for bone conservation.[22]

Smile Expression of the face in which the lip commissures are elevated to connote pleasure, approval, or joy. Act of producing a smile.[23]

Smile line Imaginary line following the contour of the upper lip in the act of smiling. The contour of the lower lip generally parallels the curvature of the incisal edges of the maxillary anterior teeth. In arranging maxillary artificial teeth, the incisal-occlusal plane parallels the smile line to project a pleasing appearance.[24,25] See also: *Lip line*.

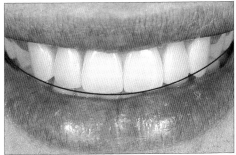

Smile line.
(Reprinted from Aiba[26] with permission.)

Socioeconomic factors Issues included when describing the relationship between financial activity and social life. For example, as a patient cost-reduction factor, the use of implants for patients with an edentulous mandible with considerable bone loss has enabled overdenture placement supported by two anterior implants to provide enhanced treatment results for this population.

Socket See: *Extraction socket*.

Socket graft See: *Bio-Col technique*.

Socket preservation See: *Extraction socket*.

Soft tissue Any noncalcified tissue. In the oral cavity, usually refers to the oral mucous membranes, including the gingiva.

Soft tissue augmentation Grafting procedure aimed at increasing soft tissue volume.

Soft tissue cast   Working cast in which the implant analog is enveloped in an elastic material simulating mucosal tissues to facilitate laboratory procedures.[4]   See also: *Implant-level impression.*

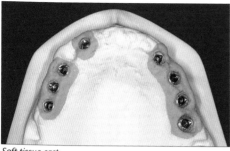

Soft tissue cast.
(Reprinted from QDT[27] with permission.)

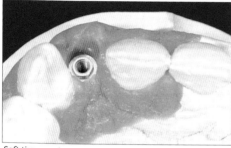

Soft tissue cast.
(Reprinted from Watzek[28] with permission.)

Soft tissue defect   Defect of soft tissue that may include scarring from previous surgeries, inadequate soft tissue margins, or inadequate soft tissue volume related to an underlying bone defect following trauma or infection.

Soft tissue graft   See also: *Soft tissue augmentation.*

Solder joint   Interface of adjacent metallic surfaces united with appropriate metal alloys to produce a continuous unit.[13,22]

Solid screw   Retentive element without an open or hollow interior bore.

Somatoprosthesis   Artificial body part.

Sounding   See: *Bone sounding.*

Spacemaking   Property of surgical site capable of maintaining a space under a membrane for the purpose of guided bone regeneration (GBR). This may be provided by: *(1)* defect morphology in either three-wall or two-wall defects; *(2)* use of bone grafts or substitutes to support the membrane; *(3)* membrane itself, which is rigid and stable enough to maintain a secluded space below; or *(4)* using a reinforced membrane to avoid membrane collapse.

Spark erosion   See: *Electric discharge method (EDM).*

Speaking space   Available distance between the incisal and/or occlusal surfaces of the teeth or trial occlusion wax rims during directed acts of speech.[22,29]   See also: *Vertical dimension.*

Specialized oral mucosa
See: *Mucosa; Oral mucosa.*

Spiral drill   Cutting instrument with a three-dimensional continuous curving surface around a shaft used to create cylindrical openings in bone.

Spirochete   General term for any microorganism of the order Spirochaetales. This spiral, gram-negative, highly motile bacterium is characterized by a flexible cell wall. It is markedly increased in number in diseased periodontal pockets. The major genus in diseased periodontal tissues is the *Treponema.*   See also: *Treponema denticola.*

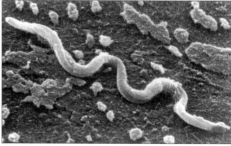

Spirochete (scanning electron micrograph; high magnification). (Reprinted from Ingraham and Ingraham[30] with pemission.)

S

Splinting   Process of stabilization via connecting teeth, implants, bars, or other prosthetic devices to create a stronger unit. Splinting may be provided by fixed or removable prostheses that are supported by natural teeth or implants. Surgical applications may involve any material or device to immobilize a body part compromised by trauma, surgery, or disease.[13,31]

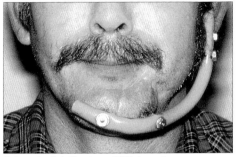

Extraoral splint. (Courtesy of W.R. Laney.)

Split-crest technique   See: *Alveolar ridge augmentation, Split-ridge technique for.*

Split-ridge technique   See: *Alveolar ridge augmentation, Split-ridge technique for.*

Split-thickness graft
See: *Subepithelial connective tissue graft.*

Spongy bone   See: *Trabecular bone.*

SPT   Abbreviation for *supportive periodontal therapy.*   See: *Periodontal maintenance.*

Square impression coping   Impression coping designed as a square when viewed in cross section. The height varies as does the manufacturer's design; it may include indentations (ie, concavities or convexities) along the length of the square.   See also: *Impression coping.*

Stability   Property of a material, implant, prosthesis, or dental restoration to maintain an intended physical position or state when subjected to forces disturbing its equilibrium; eg, resistance to displacement of a prosthesis or restoration in the horizontal plane.[22,32]   See also: *Primary stability; Secondary stability.*

Stabilization   See: *Bicortical stabilization; Bilateral stabilization.*

Stack   Vertically aligned and assembled combination of a prosthetic restoration, abutment and implant.

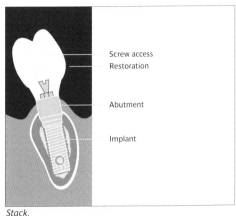

Screw access
Restoration

Abutment

Implant

Stack.
(Redrawn from Brånemark[13] with permission.)

Staged protocol
See: *Stage-one surgery; Stage-two surgery.*

Stage-one surgery   Placement of an implant with a healing screw in a submerged fashion. Followed by stage-two surgery.

Stage-two surgery   Following stage-one surgery, the uncovering or reopening of an implant site at a later date by a small gingival excision or tissue punch to remove the healing screw and replace it with an abutment.

Staggered offset   Positioning of multiple implants (minimum of three) such that the implant bodies are not in a linear relationship; the purpose is to increase the mechanical stability of the resulting assembly.   See also: *Tripodization.*

Standard abutment Prosthetic implant component meeting the recommended design for restoration. Early use of the term was specific to a particular implant company.

Standard deviation (SD) Measure of the dispersion or variability of a set of values. Defined mathematically, it is the square root of the variance of these observations. By definition, approximately 68% of the values in the normal distribution (or bell-shaped curve) fall within one SD on either side of the mean. If the SD exceeds one half the mean, the data are not normally distributed.[11] See also: *Variance*.

Standard error (SE) Measure of the dispersion of the possible differences between samples of two populations, usually the difference between the means of the samples.[11]

Standard of care Treatment that experts agree is appropriate, accepted, and widely used. Healthcare providers are obligated to provide patients with the standard of care.[34]

Staple implant See: *Transosseous implant*.

Static loading Placement of an implant into a constant loading situation. Static load is applied to an implant through a non passive or misfitting prosthesis in a multiple implant restoration. Static loading of an implant also occurs in situations where the implant is used for orthodontic anchorage. See also: *Loading*.

Statistical significance
See: *Null hypothesis; P value*.

Stem cell Primary undifferentiated cell that retains the ability to produce an identical copy of itself when divided (self-renew) and differentiated into another cell type. See also: *Hematopoietic stem cell; Mesenchymal stem cell (MSC)*.

Stent Fabricated device used surgically to maintain tissue position (eg, graft) or maintain lumen or intended defect patency. See also: *Surgical template*.

Stepped implant Specific implant shaft design that incorporates concentric steps that narrow in width toward the apex of the implant.

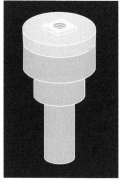

Stepped implant.

Stereognosis Ability to perceive weight and form of an object by touch.

Stereolithographic guide Surgical guides that assist placement of implants in vivo in the same locations and directions as those in a planned computer simulation.

Stereolithography Technique for creating solid plastic, three-dimensional objects from computer-aided design (CAD) drawings by selectively solidifying an ultraviolet-sensitive liquid resin (photopolymer) using a laser beam. In implant dentistry, these physical models can reproduce the true maxillary and mandibular anatomic dimensions. A stereolithography machine has four important parts: a tank filled with several gallons of liquid photopolymer, which is a clear, liquid plastic; a perforated platform immersed in the tank, which can move up and down in the tank as the printing process proceeds; an ultraviolet laser; and a computer that drives the laser and the platform. Called also *three-dimensional layering* or *three-dimensional printing*.

Sterile technique   Method of placing implants under sterile, conventional operating room conditions.

Stippling   Gingival appearance of fine light or dark dots, or a spotted appearance. It is a normal adaptive condition in which the attached gingiva presents a lobulated surface, with an orange-peel appearance.

Straight implant   See: *Parallel-sided implant.*

Strain   Deformation of a structure when external load is applied.   Compare: *Stress.*

Stress   Force per unit area.   Compare: *Strain.*

Stress bending   Load applied to a structure that tends to deform. For an implant, bending stress deforms the long axis of the implant body.   See also: *Nonaxial loading.*

Stress concentration   Area within a structure at which applied external force creates heightened internal strain. It is also the point at which a structure is more likely to fail catastrophically or through fatigue loading.

Stress distribution   The pattern of distribution of stress as seen when a load is applied to an object or series of objects. For example, the stress distribution in bone associated with an implant–supported restoration depends on the number and location of implants, the design of the prosthetic superstructure, and the anatomy of the surrounding bone.[35]

Stress shielding   Situation, particularly in orthopedic joint replacement, in which an implant is stiffer than the bone in which it is placed. Under loading the implant bears the load, and the surrounding bone undergoes disuse atrophy. The shaft of the implant shields the bone from functional loading.

Stripped thread   Screw (or an internal screw channel) that has lost its thread architecture because the screw was inserted and tightened incorrectly or because the screw was pulled from its channel without unscrewing.

Stripping   Removal of the surface of an object; the act of creating a stripped thread.   See also: *Stripped thread.*

Student *t* test   See: *t test.*

Stud-type attachment system
See: *Ball attachment system; O-ring.*

Subantral augmentation
See: *Maxillary sinus floor elevation.*

Subepithelial connective tissue graft   Graft of connective tissue taken from the palate for root coverage in instances of recession or lack of keratinized tissue. This procedure has been adopted in implant dentistry with the purpose of enhancing soft tissue contours for esthetics. The advantage of this procedure as compared to a free gingival graft is its esthetic superiority, dual blood supply, and less donor-site postoperative morbidity.[36]

Sublingual artery   The sublingual artery arises at the anterior margin of the hyoglossus and runs forward between the genioglossus and mylohyoideus to the sublingual gland. It supplies the gland and gives branches to the mylohyoideus and neighboring muscles, as well as to the mucous membrane of the floor of the mouth and lingual gingiva.[37]

Submerged healing   Implant placement with complete primary soft tissue closure, requiring a second surgical procedure to expose the implant and initiate prosthetic restoration following healing. (See figure next page.)

S

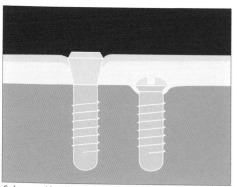

Submerged healing (right).
(Redrawn from Cochran and Mahn[38] with permission.)

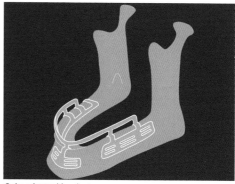

Subperiosteal implant.

Submerged implant   See: *Submerged healing.*

Subperiosteal s. i.   See: *Complete subperiosteal implant; Eposteal implant; Unilateral subperiosteal implant.*

Submergible implant   Implant that is "submerged beneath the oral mucosa at time of surgical placement."[39]   See also: *Two-stage implant placement.*

Subnasal elevation   Rarely performed surgical technique to enhance anterior bone height in the anterior maxilla. Surgically, it can be compared with a sinus floor elevation; instead of elevating the maxillary sinus membrane, the nasal mucosa is elevated.

Subperiosteal implant   Custom-fabricated implant frame to fit directly on bone. As originally designed, the fabrication procedure requires two surgical procedures, the first of which allows impressioning of the supporting bone; the second for framework placement. Framework is made in a latticework configuration to cover an extensive bony surface and can be made to incorporate permucosal posts and/or an additional, continuous bar superstructure.[40]   See also: *Eposteal implant.*

Subtracted implant surface   Implant surface created through removal of material by exposure to acid, abrasives, or electrolysis. Subtractive process generally creates roughness intended to enhance cell proliferation and osseointegration.

Subtraction radiography   Technique requiring digital imaging. Differences in gray values are stored in an image matrix and can be made visible when a baseline radiograph is subtracted from a follow-up radiograph. When the same object is exposed at least two or more times in the same way, the changes over time in hard tissue structures like bone or enamel can thus be detected. This technique permits detection of mineral loss in both enamel and bone before it is visible in conventional radiography.

Subtractive surface treatment
See: *Subtracted implant surface.*

Succedaneous dentition
See: *Dentition, Permanent.*

Success criterion   Condition established to determine whether data have satisfied their objectives and met the requirements for success.

Success rate   Percentage of patients or units that have completed a study after a specified period of time and have met defined success criteria.   See also: *Cumulative success rate.*

Sulcular epithelium   See: *Crevicular epithelium.*

Tissue punch for s. e.   See: *Implant exposure; Tissue punch technique.*

Sulcular incision   Incision that maintains the entire marginal gingival tissue. It is made from the base of the gingival sulcus, parallel to the root surface, reaching the alveolar bone crest.

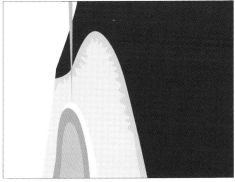

Sulcular incision.
(Redrawn from Sato[41] with permission.)

Summer osteotome technique   See: *Maxillary sinus floor elevation; Osteotome technique.*

Superstructure   Framework skeleton for the attachment of a matrix holding artificial teeth comprising the prosthesis, which is connected directly to dental implants, an infrastructure, and/or as mesostructure.[4,22] Called also *suprastructure.*

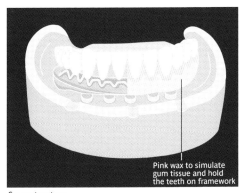

Pink wax to simulate gum tissue and hold the teeth on framework

Superstructure.
(Redrawn from Taylor and Laney[42] with permission.)

Supportive periodontal therapy (SPT)   See: *Periodontal maintenance.*

Suppuration   Formation or discharge of pus; associated with an acute or chronic infection.[43]

Surface bonding   Additive surface applied to the implant body.

Surface of implant   See: *Implant surface.*

Surface treatment   Modification to the implant surface, either structural or chemical, which alters its properties. It may be additive or subtractive in nature.   See also: *Additive surface treatment; Anodizing surface treatment; Fluoride-modifying surface treatment; Microtextured surface treatment; Oxidating surface treatment; Subtracted implant surface.*

Surgical   Any condition pertaining to or correctable by surgery.

Surgical bed   Surgically prepared site, ready to receive an implant, bone graft, or soft tissue graft.

Surgical dressing   See: *Periodontal dressing.*

Surgical guide   See: *Surgical template.*

Surgical implant   Device made from a non living material and surgically placed into the human body where it is intended to remain for a significant period of time to perform a specific function.[44]

Surgical navigation   Computer-aided intraoperative navigation of surgical instruments and operation site, using real-time matching to patients' anatomy. During surgical navigation, deviations from a preoperative plan can be immediately observed on the monitor.[45]

Surgical stage
See: *Stage-one surgery; Stage-two surgery.*

Surgical stent   See: *Stent*.

Surgical template   Laboratory-fabricated guide based on ideal prosthetic positioning of implants used during surgery. Called also *surgical guide*.

Survival rate   Percentage or estimated percentage of subjects in which a given censored event (eg, implant failure, prosthesis failure) has not occurred during a time period measured from a given starting point. It is usually used to describe the percentage of implants that remain in the mouth over a specified period of time.[11]   See also: *Kaplan-Meier analysis*.

S value   In the study of surface roughness and topography of dental implants, *S* values are measurements of irregularities in three dimensions.[46]

Symphysis   Anterior line of fusion of the two halves of the mandible, which ossifies during the first year of life.

Syngeneic graft   See: *Isograft*.

Synthetic bone material   See: *Bone substitute*.

Synthetic graft material   See: *Bone substitute*.

Systematic review   Summary of medical literature, which uses explicit methods to perform a thorough literature search and is followed by a critical appraisal of individual studies using appropriate statistical techniques to combine studies that meet defined inclusion and exclusion criteria.

S

T

Tannerella forsythensis Fusiform, fastidious, anaerobic gram-negative member of the *Cytophaga-Bacteroides* family implicated in periodontal and peri-implant diseases. *T forsythensis, Porphyromonas gingivalis,* and *Treponema denticola* form a red complex of species associated with aggressive periodontal infections. This organism, previously described as *Bacteroides forsythus,* was subsequently reclassified to *T forsythensis* based upon its phylogenetic position.

Tantalum (Ta) Malleable metal used in the past to fabricate plates, wires, and discs for implantation; atomic number 73 and atomic weight 180.948.

Tape See: *Articulating tape.*

Tapered implant Shape of an implant body when viewed in profile, lengthwise. A tapered implant usually narrows apically.

Tapered impression coping Impression coping designed to narrow toward the occlusal surface; varies in length.[1]

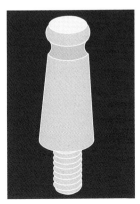
Tapered impression coping.

Tapping Final bone preparation of the screw thread configuration prior to implant placement.

Tarter See: *Calculus.*

T cell Thymus-dependent lymphocytes that are spherical cells of the lymphoid series and among the principal cells involved in the cell-mediated immune response.

TCP Abbreviation for *Tricalcium phosphate.*

Team approach Multidisciplinary combination and collaboration of care and/or therapy providers in the restorative management of a patient whose treatment involves dental implants.[2-4]

Teflon compression ring Prosthetic component made of polyoxymethylene intended to provide resilience between the implant and the prosthesis. This ring is placed between the transmucosal element and the prosthesis.[5] See also: *Intramobile connector.*

Telescopic coping Concept in fixed prosthodontics in which an intermediate coping can be designed to compensate for a malaligned retainer. Stacked crowns are fabricated with the contours to fit within the confines defined by a single restoration, without causing clinical or prosthetic complications associated with overcontoured crowns. This technique is used in overdenture therapy in which natural teeth are retained and restored using a crown (ie, telescopic coping) designed with minimal thickness to serve as a patrix component; the matrix component

T

(ie, telescopic crown) is then incorporated into the prosthesis.[6,7]

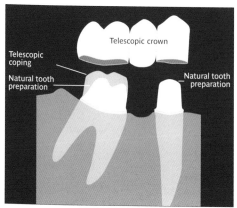

Telescopic coping.

Telescopic coping attachment system   Retentive mechanism that employs a frictional fit between the matrix and patrix components. External surface of the patrix mirrors the internal surface of the matrix and fits within the confines of the matrix for a frictional, passive fit.[8,9]   See also: *Telescopic coping.*

Template   See: *Surgical template.*

Temporary abutment   Implant component used for a limited period of time prior to fabrication of the definitive prosthesis.

Temporary cement   See: *Cement.*

Temporary cylinder   See: *Temporary abutment.*

Temporary healing cuff   See: *Healing abutment.*

Temporary prosthesis   See: *Provisional prosthesis.*

Temporomandibular articulation   Ginglymo-arthrodial-type articulating joint involved in the bilateral connection of mandibular condyles to the temporal bone. Anatomic structures comprising the joint are: the anterior part of the glenoid cavity of the temporal bone, its articular eminence, and the mandibular condyle; the lig-

aments supporting the joint are the temporomandibular, capsular, sphenomandibular, stylomandibular, and the articular disk or meniscus. The joint facilitates mandibular movements involving depression and elevation, as well as forward, backward, and lateral combinations.[10,11]

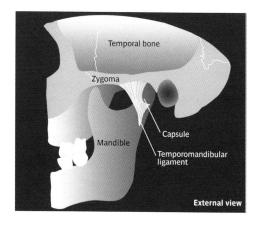

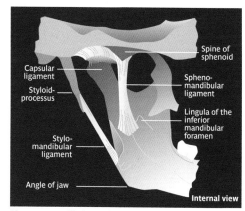

Temporomandibular articulation.
(Redrawn from Gray[12] with permission.)

Temporomandibular joint   Articulation between the mandibular condyles and glenoid fossa of the temporal bone is capable of translation and rotation movements. The disk is composed of dense fibrous connective tissue, while the posterior attachment is highly vascularized and innervated. The joint is surrounded by the capsular ligament, a fibrous capsule.   See also: *Temporomandibular articulation.*

Tensile strain
Elongation ÷ original length × 100 %.

Tensile stress   Force applied to an object that elongates or stretches.

Tension-free wound closure   Wound closure that can be obtained without flap tension. Underlying periosteum may need to be released to provide coverage of an augmented site.   See also: *Releasing incision.*

Tent pole procedure   Operation in which the anterior part of an atrophic mandible is exposed by extraoral approach; periosteum and soft tissues are elevated to expose the superior aspect of the mandible. Dental implants are placed by tenting the soft tissue matrix to prevent graft resorption. Particulate autogenous bone chips are onlayed under the periosteum and around the implants.

Tenting screw   Metal screw used in guided bone regeneration (GBR) procedures to support barrier membranes retaining space for new bone formation.[13]

Test, chi-square   See: *Chi-square test.*

Tetracycline   Group of wide-spectrum antibiotics seldom used in treatment of oral infections but may be used for rhinogenic infections. Some are natural (ie, isolated from certain species of *Streptomyces*) and others are produced semisynthetically. Tetracyclines and their analogues inhibit protein synthesis by their action on microbial ribosomes and have anti-matrix metalloproteinase (MMP) activity. All have similar toxic and pharmacologic properties, differing mainly in their absorption and suitability for various modes of administration. They are effective against a broad range of aerobic and anaerobic gram-positive and gram-negative bacteria, as well as rickettseae, chlamydiae, and mycoplasmas. Because of the binding to calcium, it is not advisable to use tetracyclines in the treatment of infections in children.

Tetracycline bone labeling   Permanent labeling of osteoid (bone matrix) as it mineralizes in a two-phase process. With up to 80% of complete mineral uptake regulated by osteoblasts, the remaining 20% is regulated by osteocytes. The osteoid zone is separated from the mineralized part of the bone by a layer called the mineralization front. This layer is able to bind tetracycline, resulting in a permanent fluorescent line.

Textured surface   See: *Rough implant surface.*

Texturing   Application of texture; to roughen.

TGF   Abbreviation for *Transforming growth factor.*

TGF-β   Abbreviation for *Transforming growth factor beta.*

Thick flat periodontium
See: *Periodontal biotype, Thick.*

Thin scalloped periodontium
See: *Periodontal biotype, Thin.*

Thread   Grooves cut into the walls of a cylinder making it a screw (positive) or a screw channel (negative). These structures guide the insertion and removal of a screw or bolt. Also, the act of inserting a screw or bolt into its receiving channel. Example: *The next step is to thread the occlusal screw into the abutment.*

Major diameter of t.   Greatest thread diameter of a tapered screw. The diameter by which the screw is designated.   Compare: *Thread, Minor diameter.*

Minor diameter of t.   Smallest thread diameter of a tapered screw.   Compare: *Thread, Major diameter.*

Thread flank   Side of a thread between the crest of the thread and the depth of the thread. In most applications the thread angle between the flanks of a thread is 60 degrees. (See figure next page.)

Thread lead   Distance between screw threads as measured in the direction of the long axis of the screw.   Compare: *Thread pitch*.

Thread pitch   Distance between threads, in millimeters, as measured perpendicularly to the thread axis. In American units, thread pitch is given in threads per inch.   Compare: *Thread lead*.

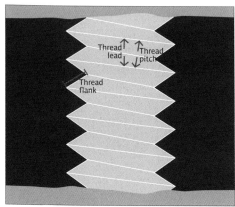

Thread flank, thread lead, thread pitch.

Threaded implant   Implant body design resembling a screw, including helical threading developed into the external surface of the implant. Term does not describe the connnection present between the anchorage component and the prosthetic component, which may or may not include an internal bore within the anchorage component.   See also: *Implant thread*.

Three-dimensional guidance system for implant placement   A computed tomography (CT) scan is performed to provide image data for a three-dimensional guidance construct for implant placement. A guide is a structure or marking that directs the motion or positioning of something, thus in implant dentistry this term should not be used as a synonym for *surgical implant guide*. A radiographic guide is rather used as a positioning device in intraoral radiography.   See also: *Radiographic prosthesis*.

Three-dimensional imaging
   See: *Stereolithography*.

Three-dimensional layering
   See: *Stereolithography*.

Three-dimensional modeling
   See: *Stereolithography*.

Three-dimensional printing
   See: *Stereolithography*.

Thrombocyte   See: *Platelet*.

Ti   Abbreviation for *Titanium*.

Tibia   Bone located medial and anterior to the fibula. The tibia articulates superiorly with the femur and patella, laterally with the fibula, and inferiorly with the ankle.[14]

Tibial bone harvest   Extraoral source of autogenous cancellous bone harvested from the lateral proximal tibia, which can be performed in an ambulatory setting under intravenous sedation. This procedure is rarely used in daily practice.[15]

Tissue   Composed of cells of a given degree of specialization, differentiation, maturation, and a characteristic intercellular substance. Although the intercellular substance may comprise the major volume, tissues are primarily classified according to the predominating types of cells they contain.

   Bone t.   Consists of 70% mineral and 30% organic material. Hydroxyapatite (HA) comprises 95% of the mineral and the other 5% comprises complex salts with magnesium, fluorine, sodium, potassium, and chlorine. The organic part consists of 98% matrix, where collagen type I comprises 95% and noncollagenous proteins 5%. The remaining 2% of organic material are the cells, osteoblasts, osteocytes, osteoclasts, and lining cells.

Soft t.   See: *Soft tissue.*

Tissue bank   Centers for acquiring, characterizing, and storing human organs or tissue for future use by other individuals. It may also designate storage of information about tissues (eg, bone bank, skin bank).

Tissue conditioner   Elastomeric material with limited flow properties used to massage abused or healing soft tissues. Usually a modified acrylic resin consisting of a polymer (eg, ethyl methacrylate or co-polymer) and an aromatic ester – ethyl alcohol mixture is often used in an existing prosthesis.[16-18]

Tissue conditioning   Process of restoring health to oral stress-bearing soft tissues following surgical or mechanical trauma using the occluding prostheses to transmit continuous stress of force and motion to the basal-seat tissues. A tissue conditioner is often used.[19]

Tissue engineering   Combination of principles of life and engineering sciences used to develop materials and methods to repair damaged, lost, or diseased tissue. It is also used to create entire tissue and organ replacements.

Tissue-integrated prosthesis   Screw-connected, fixed or removable, orodental, maxillofacial restoration retained by osseointegrated endosseous implants. Term was originally proposed by P.-I. Brånemark and colleagues (Sweden) and intended for a full-arch prosthesis fabricated for an edentulous arch.[2]

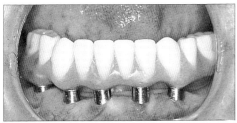

Tissue-integrated prosthesis.
(Reprinted from Branemark et al[20] with permission)

Tissue integration   Interdigitation of soft or hard tissues with an implant biomaterial.

Tissue punch   Surgical instrument used to create a circular soft tissue incision for exposing a submerged implant.

Tissue punch technique   Surgical technique to gain access to an implant following a completed healing period; removes the overlying soft tissues using a blade, disposable tissue punch, or laser. The disadvantage of this method is the loss of valuable keratinized mucosa.

Tissue recession   Drawing away of a tissue from its normal position (eg, gingival recession).   See also: *Gingival recession; Peri-implant tissue recession.*

Tissue-supported   Support of a prosthesis based entirely or partially on soft tissues overlying residual bone.[13]

Titanium (Ti)   Relatively inert and corrosion-resistant metal because of its thin (approximately 4 nm) surface oxide layer. Commercially pure, grade 4 Ti consists of more than 99% pure Ti. Ti readily absorbs proteins from biologic fluids; in contact with liquids, the surface is passivated immediately. This very stable passivity explains its corrosion resistance even against sodium chloride solutions, including physiologic saline. The pure form is not available or economical for commercial use. Ti is a relatively rare metal with anatomic number 22, atomic weight 47.90, and specific gravity of 4.5.

Commercially pure t.
   See: *Commercially pure titanium (CPTi).*

Pure t.   Elemental titanium with no impurities; not available commercially.   See also: *Commercially pure titanium (CPTi).*

T

Titanium alloy Metallic material utilized in the manufacture of endosseous implants. The most common titanium alloy used for dental implants is Ti-6Al-4V.

Titanium mesh Network of flexible interlocking titanium metal links in a fabric-like structure used to maintain created space in a bone regeneration procedure during healing. See also: *Alveolar ridge augmentation, Titanium mesh – autogenous bone grafting for*.

Titanium mesh crib, autogenous bone with See: *Alveolar ridge augmentation, Titanium mesh-autogenous bone grafting for*.

Titanium oxide Naturally occurring compounds of titanium and oxygen in various configurations. Chemical formula for titanium oxides are: TiO, TiO_2, Ti_2O_3, and Ti_3O_5. Titanium oxide occurs naturally on the surface of titanium when it is exposed to air, and it is critical to osseointegration between living bone and a titanium implant.

Titanium plasma sprayed (TPS)
See: *Plasma spray*.

Titanium reinforced Property of a material that is reinforced by a titanium structure for increased rigidity.

Titanium-reinforced expanded polytetrafluoroethylene membrane Expanded polytetrafluoroethylene (e-PTFE) membrane reinforced by an attached titanium structure that allows increased rigidity when performing guided bone regeneration (GBR) procedures.

Titanium root-form implant
See: *Endosseous implant*.

Titanium skin-penetrating implant
See: *Percutaneous implant*.

TMJ Abbreviation for *Temporomandibular joint*.

Tomography See: *Computed tomography (CT) scan; Conventional tomography*.

Tooth extraction Removal of a tooth or teeth.

Tooth fracture Breakage of natural tooth or polymer-based or ceramic prosthetic teeth.

Torque Twisting or turning force applied to an object. Specifically the force applied to an implant or screw during placement or removal. Compare: *Moment*; See also: *Cutting torque; Insertion torque; Removal torque*.

Torque controller Device that limits the potential torque that can be applied to an object; generally considered to be a safety mechanism. See also: *Torque driver*.

Torque driver Instrument used to apply torsional force to an object; generally includes a wrench and a method of gauging the torque being applied.

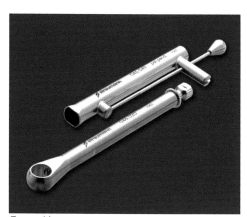
Torque driver.

Torque gauge See: *Torque indicator*.

Torque indicator Device that registers the torsional force being applied; usually registered as Newton meters, centimeters, or foot pounds. See also: *Torque driver*.

T

Torque wrench Device designed to apply a tightening force (ie, torque) with a self-limiting feature to prevent over- or undertightening. It may be manual or electric. See: *Torque driver.*

Torsion stress See: *Torque.*

Torus Bony protuberance occurring either at the midline of the palate or on the lingual aspect of the mandible.

TPS Abbreviation for *Titanium plasma sprayed.* See: *Plasma spray.*

Trabecula (pl: *trabeculae*) Supporting or anchoring strand of connective tissue, such as a strand extending from a capsule into the substance of the enclosed organ.

Trabecular bone Trabecular cancellous bone consists of bone trabeculae, thin plates or spicules with thickness ranging from 50 μm to 400 μm. Trabeculae are interconnected in a honeycomb nonending, porous system. The pattern of the trabeculae is oriented according to mechanical stress to ensure maximal adaptation to a given stress pattern. See also: *Cancellous bone.*

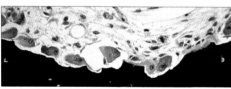
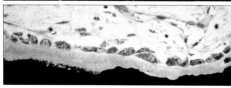
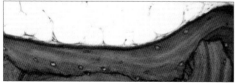

Bone remodeling of trabecular bone. (Von Kossa-McNeal; magnification x320).
(Reprinted from Buser et al[21] with permission.)

Transduction Process by which genetic material (DNA) is transmitted from one bacterial cell to another via a bacterial virus (phage), thereby changing the genetic constitution of the second organism.

Transfer coping Covering or cap used to position a die in an impression; most often made from metal or acrylic resin.[22] See also: *Coping.*

Transfer index Core or mold used to record and/or register the relative positions of teeth, anatomic structures, or implants to one another. The fabrication material is rigid and stable, so that the index can be used to transfer the three-dimensional information accurately. See also: *Index.*

Transfer jig See: *Transfer index.*

Transforming growth factor (TGF) Any of several proteins secreted by transformed cells that stimulate growth of normal cells, although not causing transformation. TGF-α (TGF-a-amino acid polypeptide, binds to the epidermal growth factor receptor (EGFR) and also stimulates growth of microvascular endothelial cells. TGF-β (TGF-beta or TGF-B) exists as several subtypes, all of which are found in hematopoietic tissue and promote wound healing.

Transforming growth factor beta (TGF-β) One of the two classes of transforming growth factors (TGF). TGF-β exists in at least three known subtypes in humans (ie, TGF-β1, TGF-β2, and TGF-β3), all of which are found in hematopoietic tissue, stimulate wound healing, and play crucial roles in tissue regeneration, cell differentiation, and embryonic development. They are upregulated in some human cancers and in vitro are antagonists of lymphopoiesis and myelopoiesis.

Transitional implant See: *Provisional implant.*

T

Transitional prosthesis Prosthetic restoration designed to facilitate the progression of patient treatment from one phase to another. Called also *conversion prosthesis*.

Transitional restoration
See: *Transitional prosthesis.*

Transmandibular implant
See: *Transosseous implant.*

Transmucosal Property of a structure extending from internal anatomic structures and communicating through the mucosa to the external environment; eg, a restored dental implant.

Transmucosal abutment Prosthetic implant component that passes through intraoral tissues (attached and/or alveolar mucosa), is accessible intraorally, and may be available as a one-piece component.[23,24]

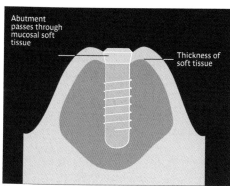

Abutment passes through mucosal soft tissue

Thickness of soft tissue

Transmucosal abutment.

Transmucosal healing See: *Nonsubmerged healing.*

Transmucosal loading Loading of an implant through the overlying soft tissue during the healing phase.

Transosseous implant Implant that is placed through the residual bone. This arch-shaped implant crosses the mandibular midline (anterior symphyseal region) and is placed into osteotomy sites in an apical-coronal direction, into the mandibular basal bone, and through the occlusal of the residual alveolar ridge using an extraoral approach.[25]

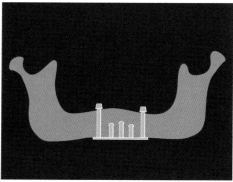

Transosseous implant.

Transosteal implant See: *Transosseous implant.*

Transport segment Alveolar segment that has been surgically prepared for alveolar distraction osteogenesis. See also: *Alveolar distraction osteogenesis.*

Trap See: *Bone trap.*

Trauma Bodily injury. Called also *injury.*

Osteoradionecrosis secondary to t. Osteoradionecrosis (ORN) that occurs in a cancer patient undergoing a radiation therapy dose greater than 70 Gy. Any trauma in the irradiated area, including the surgical trauma of implant placement, may lead to ORN because of impaired wound healing. This clinical situation is considered high risk.[26-28]

Trauma reconstruction Surgical and/or prosthetic reconstruction of the craniofacial complex, alveolar ridge, and/or teeth by means of bone grafting, implant placement, and soft tissue reconstruction.

Treatment See: *Adjunctive treatment.*

Treatment planning Organization and sequencing of treatment procedures and providers (eg, surgeons, prosthodontists) following patient diagnosis.[29]

Trephine See: *Bone trephine.*

Treponema denticola Long, thin, corkscrew-like, gram-negative, anaerobic spirochete that has been implicated as a possible etiologic agent of chronic periodontitis and peri-implantitis. Characteristic motility and morphology of the organism may be discerned by darkfield microscopy.

Trial fit gauge Replicate of an implant body used to assess the size and shape of an osteotomy.

Tricalcium phosphate (TCP) [Ca$_3$(PO$_4$)$_2$] Biodegradable bone substitute that may be used as a carrier; the biodegradation profile is unpredictable. It is similar in composition to naturally occurring bone mineral, provides an osteoconductive matrix, and is resorbed through cellular activity.

Tripodization Placement of three dental implants using a staggered offset (ie, not in a straight line) to increase resistance to nonaxial loading. See also: *Staggered offset.*

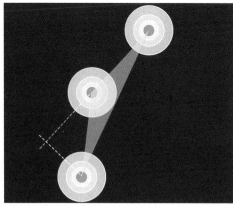

Tripodization.

Try-in Placement of a wax pattern of a tooth restoration, tooth arrangement, or any other tentative restoration in the mouth for jaw record verification, evaluation, and/or alteration prior to completion. Metal castings (eg, single-tooth restorations, frameworks, copings, or attachments) can also be placed in the mouth for evaluation of fit prior to restoration completion.[29,30]

T. of framework See: *Framework.*

T. of unglazed restoration Try-in of a ceramic or metal-ceramic restoration in the patient's mouth to evaluate contour, color, occlusion, and proximal contact tightness. The try-in is completed prior to the application of the final ceramic glaze to minimize the need for final adjustments and to create as optimal a restoration as possible.

***t* test** Statistical test often used to compare two groups on the mean value of a continuous response variable. The test is used when the variables have normal distribution. It was developed by William Gossett, a student of Karl Pearson, and published under the pseudonym Student. Called also *Student t test.*[31] See also: *Standard deviation (SD).*

Tuberosity, maxillary See: *Maxillary tuberosity.*

Tunica mucosa See: *Mucosa.*

Turned implant surface The surface texture of an implant as generated by milling machines used in manufacturing of the final implant shape. The surface is not altered subsequent to the machining process. Called also *machined implant surface.* Compare: *Polished implant surface.*

Turnover Rate at which certain biomolecules or cells are lost and/or regenerated through cell division.

T

Twist drill   Rotary cutting instrument with numerous deep spiral grooves extending from the tip to the smooth part of the shaft.[30]

Two-implant overdenture
See: *Implant overdenture.*

Two-piece implant   Anchorage component and element of the prosthetic component manufactured as two separate pieces. Implant and transmucosal abutment are assembled as separate components or elements.[32,33]

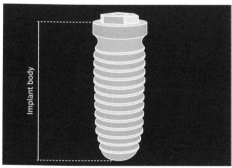

Two-piece implant (without transmucosal element).

Two-stage grafting procedures   Grafting procedures are performed when the bone defect is too large for simultaneous implant placement and sufficient primary implant stability; implant placement is delayed.   Compare: *One-stage grafting procedures.*

Two-stage implant placement   Protocol followed using two separate surgical procedures for implant placement. In the first stage, an osteotomy site is prepared, the implant is placed, and primary closure is accomplished. The second stage occurs after a specified healing period in which a soft tissue exposure is necessary to uncover the implant and allow connection to transmucosal components prior to definitive implant restoration.

Two-stage surgical approach   Category of surgical procedures that must be performed in two interventions. This group includes implant placement with submerged healing that requires a separate uncovering procedure or ridge augmentation procedures with secondary implant placement.

Type 1 bone   See: *Alveolar bone, Quality of.*

Type 2 bone   See: *Alveolar bone, Quality of.*

Type 3 bone   See: *Alveolar bone, Quality of.*

Type 4 bone   See: *Alveolar bone, Quality of.*

T

U

UCLA abutment Prosthetic implant component developed as a plastic castable pattern
that can be modified by adding wax for custom shape and dimensions. This is a founda-
tion for creating a cast-to-custom option. The
component is screw retained directly into the
implant, which circumvents the attachment
screw. [1,2] See also: *Castable abutment.*

Ultrasound stimulation Treatment modality
traditionally used in physiotherapy to treat
soft tissue disorders by deep heating tissues.
It has been used with good results in treatment of fractures or delayed union and/or
nonunions in extremities via a pulse sound
wave at 1.5 MHz with an intensity of 30 mW
per square cm. It does not seem to stimulate
healing of either defects or vertical distraction of the mandible. [3]

Underwood septum
See: *Septum, Maxillary sinus.*

Unilateral subperiosteal implant Subperiosteal implant used to restore a segment of
the arch. For example, it can be used in a partially edentulous patient requiring restoration and replacement of several teeth with
natural teeth adjacent to the partially edentulous area and on the contralateral side.
See also: *Subperiosteal implant.*

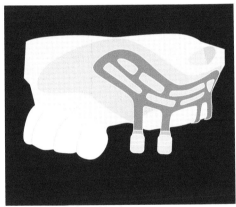

Unilateral subperiosteal implant.

Unit load Load calculated as being applied to
an individual implant within a multiple-im-
plant restoration. Also, part of the total load
on bone imposed by an endosseous implant.
Unit compression load usually equals the unit
compression stress.

U

V

Vacuum tube   See: *X-ray tube.*

Valsalva maneuver   Forceful intraoperative attempt at nasal expiration by the patient with
the nostrils held closed by the clinician to test
the possible loss of integrity of the maxillary
sinus membrane.[1]

Variance   Degree of dispersion of data about
the mean. The square root of the variance is
the standard deviation. For bell-shaped
curves, the larger the variance, the flatter the
distribution curve; the smaller the variance,
the more peaked the curve.[2]   See also: *Standard deviation (SD).*

VAS   Abbreviation for *Visual analog scale.*

Vascular endothelial growth factor (VEGF)   Peptide factor, existing in four forms with different
lengths (ie, 121, 165, 189, and 206 amino
acids) that is mitogenic for vascular endothelial cells and promotes tissue vascularization.
Its levels are elevated in hypoxia, and it is important in tumor angiogenesis.

Vascular supply   Supply of nutrients from the
vasculature to an elevated flap or surgical site.

Vascularization   See: *Angiogenesis.*

VDO   Abbreviation for *Vertical dimension of
occlusion.*

Vector   Quantity described both in magnitude
and in direction. A force vector is the application of force of a given magnitude applied in
a given direction.

Nonviral v.   See: *Gene therapy, Nonviral;
Gene transfer.*

Viral v.   See: *Gene therapy, Viral; Gene Transfer.*

VEGF   Abbreviation for *Vascular endothelial
growth factor.*

Veneer   Coating of predetermined thickness,
usually resin or ceramic, attached to a crown
restoration or pontic by bonding, cementation, or mechanical retention.[3,4]

Vent   Hole placed in an indirect restoration to
reduce seating pressure and to allow escape
of excess cement during cementation. Also a
verb explaining the act of creating the hole in
a restoration.

Verification cast   New cast made from the reassembled index of implants following the validation of fit.[5]   See also: *Verification index.*

Verification index   Assembled recording of
the positional relationship of implants made
on a cast or in the mouth for the interchangeable validation of fit. If the fit is incorrect, the
index is sectioned and reassembled.[5]

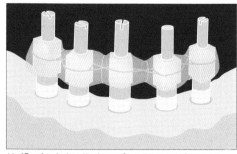

*Verification index. (Redrawn from Procera Laboratory
Manual[6] with permission.)*

Verification jig See: *Verification index.*

Vertical alveolar distraction Alveolar distraction in an apicocoronal direction. See also: *Alveolar distraction osteogenesis.*

Vertical bone height Height of the mandible in the midsagittal plane measured from the inferior border of the edentulous mandible to the top of the crest of the alveolar ridge. This measurement may also be made on a panoramic radiograph. For the maxilla, a superior landmark is defined and the height is measured from there to the crest of the residual ridge.

Vertical dimension Available distance between the incisal and/or occlusal surfaces of the teeth or trial wax occlusion rims during directed acts of speech. Called also *speaking space.*[7,8]

Vertical dimension of occlusion (VDO) Measurement between facial reference marks when the teeth or wax occlusion rims are in contact.[4] See also: *Occlusion.*

Vestibular Common reference to the trough or space between the lateral or buccal surfaces of the teeth or residual ridges and the lips and cheeks; may also refer to the trough or space between the lingual surfaces of the teeth or residual ridges and the tongue.[4]

Vestibular incision Incision placed in the buccal mucosa of the vestibulum.

Vestibuloplasty Surgical procedure that increases vestibular depth. See also: *Preprosthetic vestibuloplasty.*

Visual analog scale (VAS) Rating scale used to determine the degree of conditions or stimuli (ie, pain) a patient is experiencing. Visual analog scales represent a line with clearly defined endpoints expressing on one side of the scale the absence of stimuli (ie, no pain) while the opposite side represents the highest degree of stimuli (ie, worst pain ever). The pain or stimuli perception is marked by making a point along the defined line.[2]

Vital biomechanics Subfield of biomechanics that concerns the manner of biologic response to mechanical usage and loads as well as other physical stimuli.

Vitamin D receptor (VDR) Member of the steroid hormone receptor superfamily through which vitamin D and its analogs exert their actions. Vitamin D is a potent modulator of the immune system and involved in regulating cell proliferation and differentiation.[9]

Vitreous carbon Biocompatible carbon that is processed to reduce its brittleness. It is made from carbon containing aldehydes by a thermic degradation via high temperatures (1,000 to 3,000°C), resulting in a 99.98% pure carbon. Implants of vitreous carbon were designed and used in the 1970s; however, fibrous encapsulation without osseointegration took place. It is therefore not currently used as material for implants.

Volkmann canal Oblique channel that connects osteons to each other and the periosteum.

V-Y advancement flap Flap designed to lengthen an area of soft tissue and/or assure primary coverage without tension following tissue removal. Incision is first made in the form of a V and then sutured in the form of a Y.[10]

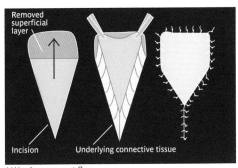
V-Y advancement flap.

W

Wax trial prosthesis   Preliminary prosthetic restoration seated in the mouth for the evaluation of maxillomandibular records, fit, and appearance.[1,2]

Waxing sleeve   Prefabricated, open-ended, castable plastic pattern (ie, coping) used for the direct shaping of contours for a restoration framework.[3,4]

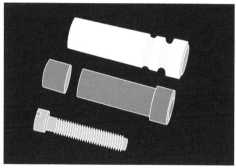

Waxing sleeve.

Waxup   Wax and/or plastic pattern contoured to the desired form for a trial denture or castable framework.[1,2]

White blood cell   See: *Leukocyte.*

Wilcoxon rank sum test   See: *Rank sum test.*

Witness   See: *Expert witness.*

Wolff Law   Principle of bone healing and/or remodeling based upon the understanding that bone remodels in response to physical stress by depositing bone in locations of increased stress and resorbing bone in areas of little or no stress.[5,6]

Working occlusion   Occluding tooth contact on the side of the arch toward which the mandible is moved.[2]

Working side   See: *Occlusion.*

Wound   Damage to living tissue; forcible interruption of the continuity of any tissue. Called also *injury* or *trauma*.

Wound closure   Approximation of mucoperiosteal or mucosal flaps at the end of a surgical procedure. Wound margins are secured by sutures.   See also: *Tension-free wound closure.*

  Sutures for w. c.   Sutures that assist in keeping flap margins well adapted to each other without tension. Varying suturing techniques may be used.

Wound dehiscence   Incomplete wound healing because of insufficient blood supply, excessive postsurgical edema, or compromised healing.

  Hyperbaric oxygen treatment for w. d.   Use of hyperbaric oxygen in cases of severely compromised wound healing.   See also: *Hyperbaric oxygen treatment (HBOT).*

Wound healing   Natural process of restoration of integrity to traumatized tissue in the body. It comprises a set of events that take place in a predictable fashion to repair the damage. These events overlap in time and are categorized into separate phases: the inflammatory, proliferative, and maturation phases.

W

Woven bone   Collagen fibrils oriented in a random or felt-like manner; primarily formed in embryos. In adults it reappears when accelerated bone formation is required (ie, healing bone). It has interlacing fibrils, numerous and large osteocytes, and a rather high mineral density. The mineralization process starts 1 to 3 days after osteoid formation.   See also: *Osteogenesis.*

Wrench   Device or tool used to apply torsional force to an object, as in tightening or loosening a screw or bolt.   See also: *Cylinder wrench.*

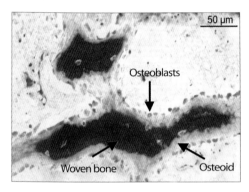

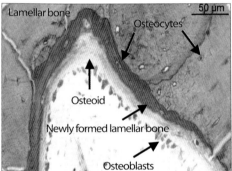

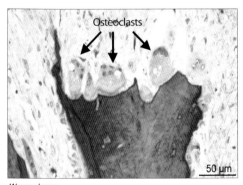

Woven bone.
(Reprinted from Watzek[7] with permission.)

X Y

Xenograft Graft taken from a donor of another species. Called also *heterograft*.

X-ray Limited part of the spectrum of electromagnetic radiation; a self-propagating transverse oscillating wave of electric and magnetic fields.

X-ray tube Vacuum tube designed to produce x-ray photons. In the tube, there is a cathode to emit electrons into the vacuum and an anode to collect the electrons, where the x-rays are produced by bremsstrahlung.

Young modulus See: *Elastic modulus.*

Z

Zirconium oxide Ceramic material used for implant components; generally attributed to have excellent mechanical properties. It is used in situations where esthetics are of primary importance and metal show-through of the tissues is a potential problem. Called also *zirconia*.

Zygomatic implant Endosseous implant placed into the zygoma as a "partial or complete alternative to bone augmentation procedures for the severely atrophic maxilla." Designed and fabricated as a long, screw-shaped implant. Implant is placed surgically using a placement appliance to help guide the position and angle of placement.[1,2] Compare: *Pterygoid implant*.

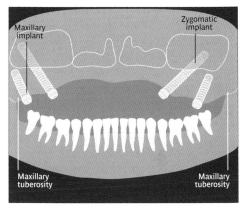

Zygomatic implant.

References

A

1. Yanase RT, Preston JD. Nomenclature for implant dentistry. In: Fonseca R, Davis WH (eds). Reconstructive and preprosthetic oral and maxillofacial surgery, 2nd ed. Philadelphia: WB Saunders Co., 1995:230 – 231.

2. Yanase RT, Preston JD. Considerations for screw/cylinder prosthetic components. In: Fonseca R, Davis WH (eds). Reconstructive and preprosthetic oral and maxillofacial surgery, 2nd ed. Philadelphia: WB Saunders Co., 1995:251, Fig 10-2.

3. Jalbout Z, Tabourian G. Glossary of implant dentistry. New Jersey: ICOI and New York University, 2004.

4. Watzek G. Endosseous implants: scientific and clinical aspects. Chicago: Quintessence Publishing Co., Inc., 1996: 377, Fig 11-35e, p 389, Fig 11-38i.

5. The American Heritage Stedman's Medical Dictionary, 2nd ed. ©2004. http://medical-dictionary.thefreedictionary.com/acute. 2007 March 7.

6. Merriam-Webster's Collegiate Dictionary, 11th ed. Springfield: Merriam-Webster, Inc., 2006. Adhesive; 15.

7. Chalian VA, Drane JB, Standish SM. Maxillofacial prosthetics. Baltimore: Williams and Wilkins Co., 1972.

8. Preiskel HW. Overdentures made easy. A guide to implant and root supported prostheses. London: Quintessence Publishing Co., Ltd., 1996:81 – 83.

9. Staubli PE, Bagley D. Attachments & implants reference manual, 2nd ed. San Mateo: Attachments International, Inc., 2002.

10. Glossary of prosthodontic terms, 8th ed. J Prosthet Dent 2005;94:1 – 81.

11. Rose LF, Mealey BL, Genco RJ, Cohen DW. Periodontics, medicine, surgery, and implants. St. Louis: CV Mosby Co., Inc., 2004.

12. Lindhe J, Karring T, Lang NP. Clinical periodontology and implant dentistry, 4th ed. Oxford: Blackwell Publishing Ltd., 2003.

13. The American Heritage Stedman's Medical Dictionary, 2nd ed. ©2004. http://medical-dictionary.thefreedictionary.com/atrophy. 2006 June 30.

14. Lekholm U, Zarb GA . Patient selection and preparation. In: Brånemark PI, Zarb GA, Albrektsson T (eds). Tissue-integrated prostheses: osseointegration in clinical dentistry. Chicago: Quintessence Publishing Co., Inc., 1985:199 – 209.

15. Watzek G. Implants in qualitatively compromised bone. London: Quintessence Publishing Co., Ltd., 2004.

16. Chin M. Distraction osteogenesis for dental implants. Atlas Oral Maxillofac Surg Clin North Am. 1999;7(1):41 – 63.

17. The anatomical basis of clinical practice. In: Standring S (ed). Gray's anatomy, 39th ed. Toronto: Churchill Livingstone, 2005.

18. Cawood JI, Howell RA. A classification of the edentulous jaws. Int J Oral Maxillofac Surg 1988;17:232 – 235.

19. Iizuka T, Smolka W, Hallermann W, Mericske-Stern R. Extensive augmentation of the alveolar ridge using autogenous calvarial split bone grafts for dental rehabilitation. Clin Oral Implants Res 2004;15(5):607 – 15.

20. Buser D, Martin W, Belser UC. Optimizing esthetics for implant restorations in the anterior maxilla: anatomic and surgical considerations. Int J Oral Maxillofac Implants 2004;19 Suppl:43 – 61.

21. Kalk WW, Raghoebar GM, Jansma J, Boering G. Morbidity from iliac crest bone harvesting. Int J Oral Maxillofac Surg 1996;54(12):1424 – 9.

22. Bloomquist DS, Feldman GR. The posterior ilium as a donor site for maxillo-facial bone grafting. Int J Oral Maxillofac Surg 1980;8(1):60 – 4.

23. Nkenke E, Weisbach V, Winckler E, Kessler P, Schultze-Mosgau S, Wiltfang J et al. Morbidity of harvesting of bone grafts from the iliac crest for preprosthetic augmentation procedures: a prospective study. Int J Oral Maxillofac Surg 2004; 33(2):157 – 63.

24. Thorwarth M, Srour S, Felszeghy E, Kessler P, Schultze-Mosgau S, Schlegel KA. Stability of autogenous bone grafts after sinus lift procedures: a comparative study between anterior and posterior aspects of the iliac crest and an intraoral donor site. Oral Surg Oral Med Oral Pathol Oral Radiol Endod 2005;100(3):278 – 84.

25. Nystrom E, Lundgren S, Gunne J, Nilson H. Interpositional bone grafting and Le Fort I osteotomy for reconstruction of the atrophic edentulous maxilla. A two-stage technique. Int J Oral Maxillofac Surg 1997;26(6):423 – 7.

26. Von Arx T, Hardt N, Wallkamm B. The TIME technique: a new method for localized alveolar ridge augmentation prior to placement of dental implants. Int J Oral Maxillofac Implants 1996;11(3):387 – 94.

27. Merck Source. Resource Library. © 2006. http://www.mercksource.com/pp/us/cns/cns_search_results.jsp. 2006 June 30.

28. Yanase RT, Preston JD. Nomenclature for implant dentistry. In: Fonseca R, Davis WH (eds). Reconstructive and preprosthetic oral and maxillofacial surgery, 2nd ed. Philadelphia: WB Saunders Co., 1995:233 – 234.

29. Lang TA, Secic M. How to report statistics in medicine. Philadelphia: American College of Physicians, 1997.

30. Yancopoulos GD, Davis S, Gale NW, Rudge JS, Wiegand SJ, Holash J. Vascular-specific growth factors and blood vessel formation. Nature 2000; 407:242 – 248.

31. Held JR, Hsu CK. Animal quality and models in biomedical research: 7th ICLAS Symposium Utrecht 1979. New York: Gustav Fischer Verlag, 1980:9 – 28.

32. Zwemer TJ. Boucher's clinical dental terminology, 4th ed. St. Louis: CV Mosby Co., Inc. 1993.

References

33 Kuzmanovic DV, Payne AG, Kieser JA, Dias GJ. Anterior loop of the mental nerve: a morphological and radiographic study. Clin Oral Implants Res 2003;14(4): 464 – 71.

34 The American Heritage Stedman's Medical Dictionary, 2nd ed. ©2004. http://medical-dictionary.thefreedictionary.com/antibiotic. 2006 June 30.

35 Dajani AS, Taubert KA, Wilson W, Bolger AF, Bayer A, Ferrieri P et al. Prevention of bacterial endocarditis: Recommendations by the American Heart Association. JAMA. 1997; 277(22):1794 – 801.

36 The American Heritage Stedman's Medical Dictionary, 2nd ed. ©2004. http://medical-dictionary.thefreedictionary.com/antrostomy. 2006 June 30.

37 Jo YH, Hobo PK, Hobo S. Freestanding and multi-unit immediate loading of the expandable implant: an up-to-40-month prospective survival study. J Prosthet Dent 2001; 85(2):148 – 55.

38 Daskalogiannakis J. Glossary of orthodontic terms. Berlin: Quintessence Publishing Co., Inc., 2000.

39 Boucher CO. Swenson's complete dentures, 6th ed. St Louis: CV Mosby Co., Inc. 1970.

40 Starcke EN, Engelmeier RL. The history of articulators: the wonderful world of grinders. J Prosthet Dent 2006;15: 131.

41 The American Heritage Stedman's Medical Dictionary, 2nd ed. ©2004. http://medical-dictionary.thefreedictionary.com/asepsis. 2006 June 30.

42 The American Heritage Stedman's Medical Dictionary, 2nd ed. ©2004. http://medical-dictionary.thefreedictionary.com/atherosclerosis. 2006 June 30.

43 Dorland's Medical Dictionary, 30th ed. Philadelphia: WB Saunders Co.; 2003. Atresia; 174.

44 The American Heritage Stedman's Medical Dictionary, 2nd ed. ©2004. http://medical-dictionary.thefreedictionary.com/atrophy. 2006 June 30.

45 Glossary of periodontal terms, 4th ed. Chicago: AAP, 2001.

46 Glossary of prosthodontic terms, 8th ed. J Prosthet Dent 2005;94(1):10 – 92.

47 Staubli PE, Bagley D. Attachments & implants reference manual. 2nd ed. San Mateo: Attachments International, Inc., 2002:266.

48 Yanase RT, Preston JD. Nomenclature for implant dentistry. In: Fonseca R, Davis WH (eds). Reconstructive and preprosthetic oral and maxillofacial surgery, 2nd ed. Philadelphia: WB Saunders Co., 1995:226, 235.

49 Yanase RT, Preston JD. Nomenclature for implant dentistry. In: Fonseca R, Davis WH (eds). Reconstructive and preprosthetic oral and maxillofacial surgery, 2nd ed. Philadelphia: WB Saunders Co., 1995:236 – 237, Fig 9-6.

50 Binon PP. Implants and components: Entering the new millennium. Int J Oral Maxillofac Implants 2000;15(1): 76 – 94.

B

1 Quirynen M, van Steenberghe D. Bacterial colonization of the internal part of two-stage implants. An in vivo study. Clin Oral Implants Res 1993 Sep;4(3):158 – 61.

2 Zwemer TJ. Boucher's clinical dental terminology, 4th ed. St. Louis: CV Mosby Co., Inc. 1993.

3 Glossary of prosthodontic terms, 8th ed. J Prosthet Dent 2005; 94:1 – 81.

4 Staubli PE, Bagley D. Attachments & implants reference manual, 2nd ed. San Mateo: Attachments International, Inc., 2002.

5 Staubli PE, Bagley D. Attachments & implants reference manual, 2nd ed. San Mateo: Attachments International, Inc., 2002:266.

6 Lindhe J, Karring T, Lang NP (eds). Clinical periodontology and implant dentistry, 3rd ed. Munksgaard, Copenhagen: 1997:Ch 19, p 577, Fig 19-34.

7 Daskalogiannakis J. Glossary of orthodontic terms. Berlin: Quintessence Publishing Co., Inc., 2000.

8 Lang NP, Araujo M, Karring T. Alveolar bone formation. In: Lindhe J, Karring T, Lang NP (eds). Clinical periodontology and implant dentistry, 4th ed. Oxford: Blackwell Publishing Ltd., 2003:867, Fig 38-1.

9 Sharry JJ. Complete denture prosthodontics, 2nd ed. New York: McGraw-Hill Book Co., Inc., 1962.

10 Iizuka T, Hallermann W, Seto I, Smolka W, Smolka K, Bosshardt DD. Bi-directional distraction osteogenesis of the alveolar bone using an extraosseous device. Clin Oral Implants Res 2005;16(6):700 – 7.

11 Sclar AG. Preserving alveolar ridge anatomy following tooth removal in conjunction with immediate implant placement. The Bio-Col technique. Atlas Oral Maxillofac Surg Clin North Am 1999;7(2):39 – 59.

12 Encarta World English Dictionary [North American Edition]. ©2006. http://encarta.msn.com/dictionary_/compatible.html. 2006 June 30.

13 Glossary of prosthodontic terms, 8th ed. J Prosthet Dent 2005;94(1):10 – 92.

14 Nevins M. Periodontal considerations in prosthodontic treatment. Curr Opin Periodontol 1993;151 – 6.

15 Merriam-Webster's Collegiate dictionary, 11th ed. Springfield: Merriam-Webster, Inc., 2006. Biomineralization; 124.

16 Garant PR. Oral cells and tissues. Chicago: Quintessence Publishing Co., Inc. 2003.

17 Tarnow D, Magner AW, Fletcher P. The effect of the distance from the contact point to the crest of bone on the presence or absence of the interproximal dental papilla. J Periodontol 1992;63(12):995 – 6.

18 Tarnow DP, Cho SC, Wallace SS. The effect of inter-implant distance on the height of inter-implant bone crest. J Periodontol 2000;71(4):546 – 9.

19 Choquet V, Hermans M, Adriaenssens P, Daelemans P, Tarnow DP, Malevez C. Clinical and radiographic evaluation of the papilla level adjacent to single-tooth dental implants. A retrospective study in the maxillary anterior region. J Periodontol 2001;72(10):1364 – 71.

20 Tarnow D, Elian N, Fletcher P, Froum S, Magner A, Cho SC et al. Vertical distance from the crest of bone to the height of the interproximal papilla between adjacent implants. J Periodontol 2003;74(12):1785 – 8.

21 Encarta World English Dictionary [North American Edition]. ©2006. http://encarta.msn.com/dictionary_/blade.html.2006 June 30.

22 Fazili M. Blade implants: presurgical preparation procedures and radiographical analyses. J Biomed Eng 1983;5(2): 141 – 4.

23 Smithloff M, Fritz ME. The use of blade implants in a selected population of partially edentulous adults. A five-year report. J Periodontal 1976;47(1):19 – 24.

180

[24] Gershkoff A. Subperiosteal and endosteal blade implants. J Prosthet Dent 1973 ;30(4):611.

[25] Burchardt H. The biology of bone graft repair. Clin Orthop Relat Res 1983;174:28–42.

[26] Von Arx T, Buser D. Horizontal ridge augmentation using autogenous block grafts and the guided bone regeneration technique with collagen membranes: a clinical study with 42 patients. Clin Oral Implants Res 2006;17(4):359–66.

[27] Buser D, Dula K, Hirt HP, Schenk RK. Lateral ridge augmentation using autografts and barrier membranes: a clinical study with 40 partially edentulous patients. Int J Oral Maxillofac Surg 1996;54(4):420–32; 432–3.

[28] Granstrom G, Tjellstrom A. The bone-anchored hearing aid (BAHA) in children with auricular malformations. Ear Nose Throat J 1997;76(4):238–240, 242, 244–247.

[29] Snik AFM, Mylanus EAM, Cremers CWRJ, Wolfaardt J, Hodgetts, WE, Somers T et al. Consensus statements on the BAHA system: where do we stand at present? Annals of Otology, Rhinology & Laryngology 2005;114(195): 1–12.

[30] Von Arx T, Cochran D, Hermann J, Schenk R, Higginbottom F, Buser D. Lateral ridge augmentation and implant placement: an experimental study evaluating implant osseointegration in different augmentation materials in the canine mandible. Int J Oral Maxillofac Implants 2001;16: 343–354.

[31] Ogiso M, Tabata T, Kuo PT, Borgese D. A histologic comparison of the functional loading capacity of an occluded dense apatite implant and the natural dentition. J Prosthet Dent 1994;71:581–588.

[32] Miyata T, Kobayashi Y, Araki H, Motomura Y, Shin K. The influence of controlled occlusal overload on peri-implant tissue: a histologic study in monkeys. Int J Oral Maxillofac Implants 1998;13:677–683.

[33] Hurzler MB, Quinones CR, Kohal RJ, Rohde M, Strub J, Teuscher U, Caffesse R. Changes in peri-implant tissue subjected to orthodontic forces and ligature breakdown in monkeys. J Periodontol 1998;69:396–404.

[34] Heitz-Mayfield L, Schmid B, Weigel C, Gerber S, Bosshardt D, Jonsson J et al. Does excessive occlusal load affect osseointegration? An experimental study in the dog. Clin Oral Implants Res 2004;15:259–268.

[35] Isidor F. Loss of osseointegration caused by occlusal load of oral implants. A clinical and radiographic study in monkeys. Clin Oral Implants Res 1996;7:143–152.

[36] Buser D, Dahlin C, Schenk RK. Guided bone regeneration in implant dentistry. Chicago: Quintessence Publishing Co., Inc., 1994:63, Fig 3-12a, 3-12b, 3-12c, 3-13, 3-14.

[37] Matsumoto H, Ochi M, Abeko Y, Hirose Y, Kaku T, Sakaguchi K. Pulsed electromagnetic fields promote bone formation around dental implants inserted into the femur of rabbits. Clin Oral Implants Res 2000;11:354–360.

[38] Rateitschack KH, Rateitschack EM, Wolf HF. Atlas de Médecine Dentaire – Paradontologie. Paris: Médecine-Sciences Flammarion, 1985: Fig 132.

[39] Brunski JB, Hurley E. Implant supported partial prostheses: biomechanical analysis of failed cases. BED Vol 29, 1995 Bioengineering Conference, Hochmuth RM, Langrana NA, Hefzy MS (eds); ASME 1995;447–448.

[40] Zwemer TJ. Boucher's clinical dental terminology, 4th ed. St Louis: CV Mosby, 1993.

[41] Araujo MG, Lindhe J. Dimensional ridge alterations following tooth extraction. An experimental study in the dog. J Clin Periodontol 2005;32(2):212–8.

[42] Lindhe J, Karring T, Lang NP (eds). Clinical periodontology and implant dentistry, 3rd ed. Munksgaard, Copenhagen: 1997:46, Fig 1-55, 1-74.

C

[1] Marchack CB, Yamashita T. Fabrication of a digitally scanned, custom-shaped abutment: a clinical report. J Prosthet Dent 2001;85(2):113–5.

[2] Zwemer TJ. Boucher's clinical dental terminology, 4th ed. St. Louis: CV Mosby Co., Inc. 1993.

[3] Glossary of prosthodontic terms, 8th ed. J Prosthet Dent 2005;94:1–81.

[4] Thomas MV, Puleo DA, Al-Sabbagh M. Calcium sulfate: a review. J Long Term Eff Med Implants 2005;15(6):599–607.

[5] Glossary of periodontal terms, 4th ed. Chicago: AAP, 2001.

[6] The American Heritage Stedman's Medical Dictionary, 2nd ed. ©2004. http://medical-dictionary.thefreedictionary.com/callus. 2006 June 30.

[7] Glossary of prosthodontic terms, 8th ed. J Prosthet Dent 2005;94:20.

[8] Merriam-Webster's Collegiate Dictionary, 11th ed. Springfield: Merriam-Webster, Inc., 2006. Cantilever;181.

[9] Watzek G. Endosseous implants: scientific and clinical aspects. Chicago: Quintessence Publishing Co., Inc., 1996.

[10] Luyten FP. Osteonal and hemi-osteonal remodeling: the spatial and temporal framework for signal traffic in adult human bone. Int J Biochem Cell Biol 1997;29(11):1241–44.

[11] Lindhe J, Karring T, Lang NP (eds.). Clinical periodontology and implant dentistry, 4th ed. Oxford: Blackwell Publishing Ltd., 2003.

[12] Lang TA, Secic M. How to report statistics in medicine. Philadelphia: American College of Physicians, 1997.

[13] Glossary of prosthodontic terms, 8th ed. J Prosthet Dent 2005;94:21.

[14] Cawood JI, Howell RA. A classification of the edentulous jaws. Int J Oral Maxillofac Surg 1988:17;232–236.

[15] Boos RH. Basic anatomic factors of jaw position. J Prosthet Dent 1954;4:200.

[16] Boucher CO. Occlusion in prosthodontics. J Prosthet Dent 1953;3:633–656.

[17] Lang LA, Sierraalta M, Hoffensperger M, Wang RF. Evaluation of the precision of fit between the Procera custom abutment and various implant systems. Int J Oral Maxillofac Implants 2003;18(5):652–8.

[18] Heydecke G, Sierraalta M, Razzoog ME. Evolution and use of aluminum oxide single-tooth implant abutments: a short review and presentation of two cases. Int J Prosthodont 2002;15(5):488–93.

[19] Encarta World English Dictionary [North American Edition]. ©2006. http://encarta.msn.com/dictionary_/cervix.html. 2006 June 30.

[20] Daskalogiannakis J. Glossary of orthodontic terms. Berlin: Quintessence Publishing Co., Inc., 2000.

[21] Terkla LG, Laney WR. Partial dentures, 3rd ed. St. Louis: CV Mosby Co., Inc. 1963: 313.

[22] Van Waas MAJ, Geertman ME, Spanjaards SG, Boerrigter EM. Construction of a clinical implant performance scale for implant systems with overdentures with the Delphi method. J Prosthet Dent 1997;77:503–9.

References

23 Brudvik JS. Advanced removable partial dentures. Chicago: Quintessence Publishing Co., Inc., 1999.

24 MedicineNet.com. MedTerms Dictionary. ©1996-2006. http://www.medterms.com/script/main/art.asp?articlekey=24051. 2006 June 30.

25 Taylor TD. Clinical maxillofacial prosthetics. Chicago: Quintessence Publishing Co., Inc., 2000.

26 Watzek G. Implants in qualitatively compromised bone. London: Quintessence Publishing Co., Ltd., 2004.

27 Kopp KC, Koslow AH, Abdo OS. Predictable implant placement with a diagnostic/surgical template and advanced radiographic imaging. J Prosthet Dent 2003;89:611–615.

28 Encarta World English Dictionary [North American Edition]. ©2006. http://encarta.msn.com/dictionary_/configuration.html. 2006 June 30.

29 Chin M. Distraction osteogenesis for dental implants. Atlas Oral Maxillofac Surg Clin North Am 1999; 7(1):41–63.

30 Shillingburg HT, Hobo S, Whitsett LD, Jacobi R, Brackett SE. Fundamentals of fixed prosthodontics, 3rd ed. Chicago: Quintessence Publishing Co., Inc., 1997.

31 Glossary of prosthodontic terms, 8th ed. J Prosthet Dent 2006;94(1):27.

32 Buser D, Dahlin C, Schenk RK. Guided bone regeneration in implant dentistry. Chicago: Quintessence Publishing Co., Inc., 1994:52, Fig 3-1.

33 The American Heritage Stedman's Medical Dictionary, 2nd ed. ©2004. http://medical-dictionary.thefreedictionary.com/cranial+bone. 2006 June 30.

34 Jalbout Z, Tabourian G. Glossary of implant dentistry. New Jersey: ICOI and New York University, 2004.

35 McGivney GP, Castleberry DJ. McCracken's removable partial prosthodontics, 8th ed. St. Louis: CV Mosby Co., Inc. 1989:37.

36 Boucher CO. Swenson's complete dentures, 6th ed. St. Louis: CV Mosby Co., Inc. 1970.

37 MedicineNet.com. MedTerms Dictionary. ©1996-2006. http:// www.medterms.com/script/main/art.asp?articlekey=2874. 2006 June 30.

38 Brånemark PI, Zarb GA, Albrektsson T. Tissue-integrated prostheses-osseointegration in clinical dentistry. Chicago: Quintessence Publishing Co., Inc., 1985:37.

D

1 Glossary of prosthodontic terms, 8th ed. J Prosthet Dent 2005;94:1–81.

2 Zwemer TJ. Boucher's clinical dental terminology, 4th ed. St. Louis: CV Mosby Co., Inc. 1993.

3 Gray H. Gray's anatomy, 15th ed. New York: Barnes and Noble, 1995.

4 The American Heritage Stedman's Medical Dictionary, 2nd ed. Boston: Houghton Mifflin Company, 2004. Dermal graft; 218.

5 Taylor TD. Clinical maxillofacial prosthetics, Chicago: Quintessence Publishing Co., Inc., 2000.

6 Diabetes and periodontal diseases. Committee on Research, Science and Therapy. American Academy of Periodontology. J Periodontol 2000;71(4):664–78.

7 Mealey BL. Periodontal implications: medically compromised patients. Ann Periodontol 1996;1:256–321.

8 Jalbout Z, Tabourian G. Glossary of implant dentistry. New Jersey: ICOI and New York University, 2004.

9 Scortecci G. Immediate function of cortically anchored disk-design implants without bone augmentation in moderately to severely resorbed completely edentulous maxillae. J Oral Implantol 1999; 25(2):70–79.

10 Daskalogiannakis J. Glossary of orthodontic terms, Berlin: Quintessence Publishing Co., Inc., 2000.

11 Schenk RJ, Hjorting-Hansen R, Buser, D. Bone integration of implants. Forum implantologicum 2006;2:14–23:15, Fig 2.

12 Chin M. Distraction osteogenesis for dental implants. Atlas Oral Maxillofac Surg Clin North Am 1999; 7(1):41–63.

13 Preiskel HW. Overdentures made easy. A guide to implant and root supported prostheses. London: Quintessence Publishing Co., Ltd., 1996.

14 Brewer AA, Morrow RM. Overdentures. St. Louis: CV Mosby Co., Inc. 1975.

E

1 Nemcovsky CE, Artzi Z, Moses O, Gelernter I. Healing of marginal defects at implants placed in fresh extraction sockets or after 4-6 weeks of healing. A comparative study. Clin Oral Implants Res 2002;13(4):410–9.

2 Aparicio C, Rangert B, Sennerby L. Immediate/early loading of dental implants: a report from the Sociedad Espanola de Implants World Congress meeting in Barcelona, Spain, 2002. Clin Imp Dent Rel Res 2003;5:57–60.

3 Encarta World English Dictionary [North American Edition]. ©2006. http://encarta.msn.com/dictionary_/element.html. 2006 June 30.

4 Yanase RT, Preston JD. Nomenclature for implant dentistry. In: Fonseca R, Davis WH (eds). Reconstructive and preprosthetic oral and maxillofacial surgery, 2nd ed. Philadelphia: WB Saunders Co., 1995:227–236.

5 Yanase RT, Preston JD. Nomenclature for implant dentistry. In: Fonseca R, Davis WH (eds). Reconstructive and preprosthetic oral and maxillofacial surgery, 2nd ed. Philadelphia: WB Saunders Co., 1995:238.

6 Jalbout Z, Tabourian G. Glossary of implant dentistry. New Jersey: ICOI and New York University, 2004.

7 Yanase RT, Preston JD. Nomenclature for implant dentistry. In: Fonseca R, Davis WH (eds). Reconstructive and preprosthetic oral and maxillofacial surgery, 2nd ed. Philadelphia: WB Saunders Co., 1995:225–249.

8 Garant PD. Oral cells and tissues. Chicago: Quintessence Publishing Co., Inc., 2003:322.

9 Strock AE, Strock MS. Method of reinforcing pulpless anterior teeth - preliminary report. J Oral Surg 1943;1:252–255.

10 Glossary of prosthodontic terms, 8th ed. J Prosthet Dent 2005;94(1):35.

11 Small IA. Metal implants and the mandibular staple bone plate. J Oral Surg 1975;33:571–578.

12 Small IA. Metz H, Kobernick S. The mandibular staple implant for the atrophic mandible. J Biomed Mater Res 1974;8(4):365–371.

13 Staubli PE, Bagley D. Attachments & implants reference manual, 2nd ed. San Mateo: Attachments International, Inc., 2002:275.

[14] Liew A, Barry F, O'Brien T. Endothelial progenitor cells: diagnostic and therapeutic considerations. Bioessays 2006; 28:261 – 70.

[15] Berman I. Color atlas of basic histology, 2nd ed. Stamford: Appleton & Lange, 1998: Ch 11, p 141, Fig 11-14.

[16] Dorland's Medical Dictionary, 30th ed. Philadelphia: WB Saunders Co.; 2003:670.

[17] Worthington P, Brånemark PI. Advanced osseointegration surgery-applications in the maxillofacial region. Chicago: Quintessence Publishing Co., Inc., 1992.

[18] Buser D, Martin W, Belser UC. Optimizing esthetics for implant restorations in the anterior maxilla: anatomic and surgical considerations. Int J Oral Maxillofac Implants 2004;19: 43 – 61.

[19] Garber DA, Belser UC. Restoration-driven implant placement with restoration-generated site development. Compend Contin Educ Dent 1995;16(8):798 – 804.

[20] Zwemer TJ. Boucher's clinical dental terminology, 4th ed. St. Louis: CV Mosby Co., Inc. 1993.

[21] Glossary of prosthodontic terms, 8th ed. J Prosthet Dent 2005; 94:36.

[22] Hammerle CH, Jung RE. Bone augmentation by means of barrier membranes. Periodontol 2000 2003;33:36 – 53.

[23] Banerjee A. Medical statistics made clear: an introduction to basic concepts. London: The Royal Society of Medicine Press Ltd., 2003.

[24] Yanase RT, Preston JD. Considerations for screw/cylinder prosthetic components. In: Fonseca R, Cavis WH (eds). Reconstructive and preprosthetic oral and maxillofacial surgery, 2nd ed. Philadelphia: WB Saunders, 1995:250 – 255.

[25] Binon PP. Implants and components: entering the new millennium. Int J Oral Maxillofac Implants 2000; 15(1): 76 – 94.

[26] Sato N. Periodontal surgery - a clinical atlas. Carol Stream: Quintessence Publishing Co., Inc., 2000:25, Fig 1-8.

F

[1] Zwemer, TJ. Boucher's clinical dental terminology, 4th ed. St. Louis: CV Mosby Co., Inc. 1993:114.

[2] Glossary of prosthodontic terms, 8th ed. J Prosthet Dent 2005;94:37.

[3] Sharry JJ. Complete denture prosthodontics, 2nd ed. New York: McGraw-Hill Book Co., Inc., 1962:228.

[4] Glossary of prosthodontic terms, 8th ed. J Prosthet Dent 2005;94:1 – 81.

[5] Chalian VA, Drane JB, Standish SM. Maxillofacial prosthetics. Baltimore: Williams and Wilkins Co., 1972.

[6] Merriam-Webster's Collegiate Dictionary, 11th ed. Springfield: Merriam-Webster, Inc., 2006. Facial symmetry; 1266.

[7] Lang NP, Araujo M, Karring T. Alveolar bone formation. In: Lindhe J, Karring T, Lang NP (eds). Clinical periodontology and implant dentistry, 4th ed. Oxford: Blackwell Publishing Ltd., 2003:869, Fig 38-3b, 38-3c.

[8] Clark, RAF. Wound repair. Curr Opin Cell Biol 1998;1: 1000 – 8.

[9] Yanase RT, Preston, JD. Nomenclature for implant dentistry. In: Fonseca R, Davis WH (eds). Reconstructive and preprosthetic oral and maxillofacial surgery, 2nd ed. Philadelphia: WB Saunders Co., 1995:239.

[10] Glossary of periodontal terms, 3rd ed. Chicago: AAP, 1992.

[11] Brånemark PI, Zarb GA, Albrektsson T. Tissue-integrated prostheses: osseointegration in clinical dentistry. Chicago: Quintessence Publishing Co., Inc., 1985.

[12] Lang TA, Secic M. How to report statistics in medicine. Philadelphia: American College of Physicians, 1997.

[13] MedicineNet.com. MedTerms Dictionary. ©1996-2006. http://www.medterms.com/script/main/art.asp?articlekey=3469. 2006 June 30.

[14] Yanase RT, Preston JD. Nomenclature for implant dentistry. In: Fonseca R, David WH (eds). Reconstructive and preprosthetic oral and maxillofacial surgery, 2nd ed. Philadelphia: WB Saunders Co., 1995:236.

[15] Zwemer TJ. Boucher's clinical dental terminology, 4th ed. St. Louis: CV Mosby Co., Inc. 1993.

[16] Taylor TD, Laney WR. Dental implants: are they for me? Chicago: Quintessence Publishing Co., Inc., 1993.

[17] Takei HH, Azzi RA. Periodontal plastic and esthetic surgery. In: Newman MG, Takei HH, Carranza FA (eds). Carranza's clinical periodontology, 9th ed. Philadelphia: WB Saunders Co., 2002:16 – 35.

[18] Ito T, Johnson JD. Color atlas of periodontal surgery. Barcelona: Espax, S.A. Publicaciones Medicas, 1994: Ch 10, p 232, Fig 10-201, p 237, Fig 10-218.

[19] Schroeder A, Zypen E, Stich H, Sutter F. The reactions of bone, connective tissue, and epithelium to endosteal implants with titanium-sprayed surfaces. Int J Oral Maxillofac Surg 1981:9:15 – 25.

G

[1] Mulligan RC. The basic science of gene therapy. Science 1993;260:926 – 32.

[2] Partridge KA, Oreffo OC. Gene delivery in bone tissue engineering: progress and prospects using viral and nonviral strategies. Tissue Engineering 2004; 10(1/2): 295 – 307.

[3] Lindhe J, Karring T, Araujo M. Anatomy of the periodontium. In: Lindhe J, Karring T, Lang NP (eds). Clinical periodontology and implant dentistry, 4th ed. Oxford: Blackwell Publishing Ltd., 2003:3 – 49.

[4] Genco RJ, Goldman HM, Cohen DW. Contemporary periodontics. St Louis: CV Mosby Co., Inc. 1990: Ch 1, p 4, Fig 1-1.

[5] Glossary of periodontal terms, 4th ed. Chicago: AAP, 2001.

[6] Uitto VJ. Gingival crevicular fluid – an introduction. Periodontol 2000 2003; 31:9-11, p 10, Fig 1.

[7] Carranza FA, Hogan EL. Gingival enlargement. In: Newman MG, Takei HH, Carranza FA (eds). Carranza's clinical periodontology, 9th ed. Philadelphia: WB Saunders Co., 2002: 16 – 35.

[8] Langer B. The esthetic management of dental implants. In: Nevins M, Mellonig JT (eds). Implant therapy. Clinical approaches and evidence of success. Volume 2. Chicago: Quintessence Publishing Co., Inc., 1998: Ch 16, p 222, Fig 16-1, 16-4d.

[9] Miller PD. A classification of marginal tissue recession. Int J Periodont Rest Dent 1985; 85(2):9 – 13.

[10] Lindhe J, Karring T, Lang NP (eds). Clinical periodontology and implant dentistry, 4th ed. Oxford: Blackwell Publishing Ltd., 2003: Ch 25, p 521, Fig 25-4.

[11] Daskalogiannakis J. Glossary of orthodontic terms. Berlin: Quintessence Publishing Co., Inc., 2000.

References

[12] Glossary of prosthodontic terms, 8th ed. J Prosthet Dent 2005;94:1 – 81.

[13] Yanase RT, Preston JD: Nomenclature for implant dentistry. In: Fonseca R, Davis WH (eds). Reconstructive and preprosthetic oral and maxillofacial surgery, 2nd ed. Philadelphia: WB Saunders Co., 1995:235.

H

[1] Preiskel HW. Overdentures made easy. A guide to implant and root supported prostheses. London: Quintessence Publishing Co., Ltd., 1996.

[2] Glossary of prosthodontic terms, 8th ed. J Prosthet Dent 2005;94:1 – 81.

[3] Boucher CO. Swenson's complete dentures, 6th ed. St. Louis: CV Mosby Co., Inc. 1970.

[4] Lang TA, Secic M. How to report statistics in medicine. Philadelphia: American College of Physicians, 1997.

[5] Winslow T, Kibiuk L. © 2001. http://stemcells.nih.gov/info/ scireport/chapter5.asp. 2007 June 20.

[6] Merriam-Webster's Collegiate Dictionary, 11th ed. Springfield: Merriam-Webster, Inc., 2006. Hex; 584.

[7] Jalbout Z, Tabourian G. Glossary of implant dentistry. New Jersey: ICOI and New York University, 2004.

[8] Simon H, Yanase RT. Terminology for implant prostheses. Int J Oral Maxillofac Implants 2003;18:539 – 543.

[9] Granstrom G. Radiotherapy, osseointegration and hyperbaric oxygen therapy. Periodontol 2000 2003;33:145 – 62.

[10] Zwemer TJ. Boucher's clinical dental terminology, 4th ed. St. Louis: CV Mosby Co., Inc. 1993.

[11] Padbury AD Jr, Tosum TF, Taba M Jr et al. The impact of primary hyperparathyroidism on the oral cavity. J Clin Endocrinol Metab 2006;91(9):3439 – 45.

I

[1] The American Heritage Stedman's Medical Dictionary, 2nd ed. ©2004. http://medical-dictionary.thefreedictionary.com/ iliac+crest. 2006 June 30.

[2] Verstreken K, van Cleyenbreugel J, Marchal G, Naert I, Suetens P, van Steenberghe D. Computer-assisted planning of oral implant surgery: a three-dimensional approach. Int J Oral Maxillofac Implants 1996;11:806 – 810.

[3] Casap N, Wexler A, Persky N, Schneider A, Lustmann J. Navigation surgery for dental implants: assessment of accuracy of the image guided implantology system. Int J Oral Maxillofac Surg 2004;62(2):116 – 119.

[4] Casap N, Kreiner B, Wexler A, Kohavi D. Flapless approach for removal of bone graft fixing screws and placement of dental implants using computerized navigation: a technique and case report. Int J Oral Maxillofac Implants 2006; 21:314 – 319.

[5] Aparicio C, Rangert B, Sennerby L. Immediate/early loading of dental implants: a report from the Sociedad Espanola de Implants World Congress meeting in Barcelona, Spain, 2002. Clin Imp Dent Rel Res 2003;5:57 – 60.

[6] Jalbout Z, Tabourian G. Glossary of implant dentistry. New Jersey: ICOI and New York University, 2004.

[7] Glossary of prosthodontic terms, 8th ed. J Prosthet Dent 2005;94:1 – 81.

[8] Zwemer, JT. Boucher's clinical dental terminology, 4th ed. St. Louis: CV Mosby Co., Inc. 1993.

[9] Encarta World English Dictionary [North American Edition]. ©2006. http://encarta.msn.com/dictionary_/implant.html. 2006 June 30.

[10] Merriam-Webster's Collegiate Dictionary, 11th ed. Springfield: Merriam-Webster, Inc., 2006. Implant; 624.

[11] Daskalogiannakis J. Glossary of orthodontic terms, Berlin: Quintessence Publishing Co., Inc., 2000.

[12] Rieger MR, Mayberry M, Brose MO. Finite element analysis of six endosseous implants. J Prosthet Dent 1990;63(6): 671 – 676.

[13] Niznick GA. A multimodal approach to implant prosthodontics. Dent Clin North Am 1989;33(4):869 – 78.

[14] Yanase RT, Preston JD. Nomenclature for implant dentistry. In: Fonseca R, Davis WH (eds). Reconstructive and preprosthetic oral and maxillofacial surgery, 2nd ed. Philadelphia: WB Saunders Co., 1995:225 – 249.

[15] Encarta World English Dictionary [North American Edition]. ©2006. http://encarta.msn.com/dictionary_/component. html. 2006 June 30.

[16] Yanase RT, Preston JD. Nomenclature for implant dentistry. In: Fonseca R, Davis WH (eds). Reconstructive and preprosthetic oral and maxillofacial surgery. 2nd ed. Philadelphia: WB Saunders Co., 1995:227.

[17] Brånemark PI, Zarb GA, Albrektsson T. Tissue-integrated prostheses: osseointegration in clinical dentistry. Chicago: Quintessence Publishing Co., Inc., 1985:12.

[18] Taylor T. Osteogenesis of the mandible associated with implant reconstruction. Int J Oral Maxillofac Implants 1989;4: 227 – 231, Fig 10, 11, 12.

[19] Hobo S, Ichida E, Garcia LT. Osseointegration and occlusal rehabilitation. Tokyo: Quintessence Publishing Co., Inc., 1990:114 – 115.

[20] Jansson S. The implant neck: smooth or provided with retention elements. A biomechanical approach. Clin Oral Impl Res 1999:10:394 – 405.

[21] Brudvik JS. Advanced removable partial dentures. Chicago: Quintessence Publishing Co., Inc., 1999:133.

[22] Quirynen M, Vogels R, Alsaadi G, Naert I, Jacobs R, van Steenberghe D. Predisposing conditions for retrograde periimplantitis, and treatment suggestions. Clin Oral Implants Res 2005;16(5):599 – 608.

[23] Granstrom G. Osseointegration in irradiated cancer patients: an analysis with respect to implant failures. Int J Oral Maxillofac Surg 2005;63(5):579 – 85.

[24] Yanase RT, Preston JD. Nomenclature for implant dentistry. In: Fonseca R, Davis WH (eds). Reconstructive and preprosthetic oral and maxillofacial surgery, 2nd ed. Philadelphia: WB Saunders Co., 1995:226 – 227.

[25] Broggini N, McManus LM, Hermann JS, Medina R, Schenk RK, Buser D, Cochran DL. Peri-implant inflammation defined by the implant-abutment interface. J Dent Res. 2006; 85(5):473 – 8.

[26] Keller JC, Stanford CM, Wightman JP, Draughn RA, Zaharias R. Characterization of titanium implant surfaces. J Biomed Mater Res 1994;28:939 – 946.

[27] Kohles SS, Clark MB, Brown CA, Kenealy JN. Direct assessment of profilometric roughness variability from typical implant surface types. Int J Oral Maxillofac Implants 2004;19:510 – 516.

[28] Merriam-Webster's Collegiate Dictionary, 11th ed. Springfield: Merriam-Webster, Inc., 2006. Implant system; 1269.

29 Shigley JE, Mischke CR. Standard handbook of machine design, 2nd ed. New York: McGraw-Hill, 1996:21.1 – 5.
30 Lang LA, Kang B, Want RF, Lang BR. Finite element analysis to determine implant preload. J Prosthet Dent 2003;90(6): 539 – 546.
31 Yanase RT, Preston JD. Nomenclature for implant dentistry. In: Fonseca R, Davis WH (eds). Reconstructive and preprosthetic oral and maxillofacial surgery, 2nd ed. Philadelphia: WB Saunders Co., 1995:225 – 227.
32 Obeid YE, Driscoll CF, Prestipino VJ. An alternative technique for an accurate implant-retained prosthesis impression. J Prosthodont 1999;8(3):160 – 2.
33 Yanase RT, Preston JD. Nomenclature for implant dentistry. In: Fonseca R, Davis WH (eds). Reconstructive and preprosthetic oral and maxillofacial surgery, 2nd ed. Philadelphia: WB Saunders Co., 1995:232.
34 Lang TA, Secic M. How to report statistics in medicine. Philadelphia: American College of Physicians, 1997.
35 Werner H, Katz J. The emerging role of the insulin-like growth factors in oral biology. J Dent Res 2004, 83:823 – 36.
36 Sato N. Periodontal surgery - a clinical atlas. Chicago: Quintessence Publishing Co., Inc., 2000:25, Fig 1-8.
37 Merriam-Webster's Collegiate Dictionary, 11th ed. Springfield: Merriam-Webster, Inc., 2006. Interproximal space; 654.
38 Chen D, Zhao M, Mundy, GR. Bone morphogenetic proteins. Growth Factors 2004;22:233 – 241.
39 The American Heritage Stedman's Medical Dictionary, 2nd ed. ©2004. http://medical-dictionary.thefreedictionary.com/syngraft. 2006 June 30.

J

1 Glossary of prosthodontic terms, 8th ed. J Prosthet Dent 2005;94(1):47.
2 Lindhe J, Karring T, Lang NP (eds.). Clinical periodontology and implant dentistry, 4th ed. Oxford: Blackwell Publishing Ltd., 2003: Ch 1, p 8 – 9, Fig 1-14a, 1-14b.

K

1 Lang TA, Secic M. How to report statistics in medicine. Philadelphia: American College of Physicians, 1997.
2 Grant DA, Stern IB, Listgarten MA. Periodontics in the tradition of Gottlieb and Orban. 6th ed. St Louis: CV Mosby Co., Inc. 1988.
3 Cawood JI, Howell RA. A classification of the edentulous jaws. Int J Oral Maxillofac Surg 1988:17:232 – 236.
4 Sethi A, Kaus T. Practical implant dentistry. London: Quintessence Publishing Co., Ltd. 2005.

L

1 Yanase RT, Preston JD. Nomenclature for implant dentistry. In: Fonseca R, Davis WH (eds). Reconstructive and preprosthetic oral and maxillofacial surgery, 2nd ed. Philadelphia: WB Saunders Co., 1995:233.

2 Yanase RT, Preston JD. Nomenclature for implant dentistry. In: Fonseca R, Davis WH (eds). Reconstructive and preprosthetic oral and maxillofacial surgery, 2nd ed. Philadelphia: WB Saunders Co., 1995:236.
3 Buser D, Dahlin C, Schenk R.K. Guided bone regeneration in implant dentistry. Chicago: Quintessence Publishing Co., Inc. 1994:52, Fig 3-5.
4 Jalbout Z, Tabourian G. Glossary of implant dentistry. New Jersey: ICOI and New York University, 2004.
5 Boyne PJ, James RA. Grafting of the maxillary sinus floor with autogenous marrow and bone. J Oral Surg 1980;38(8): 613 – 6.
6 Tatum H Jr. Maxillary and sinus implant reconstructions. Dent Clin North Am 1986;30(2):207 – 29.
7 Daskalogiannakis J. Glossary of orthodontic terms. Berlin: Quintessence Publishing Co., Inc., 2000:210.
8 Pagano M, Gauvreau K. Principles of biostatistics, 2nd ed. Pacific Grove: Duxbury, 2000.
9 Merriam-Webster's Collegiate Dictionary, 11th ed. Springfield: Merriam-Webster, Inc., 2006. Lingual; 724.
10 Garant PD. Oral cells and tissues. Chicago: Quintessence Publishing Co., Inc., 2003:200.
11 Zwemer TJ. Boucher's clinical dental terminology, 4th ed. St. Louis: CV Mosby Co., Inc. 1993.
12 Skalak R. Biomechanical considerations in osseointegrated prostheses. J Prosthet Dent 1983;49:843 – 848.
13 Lang TA, Secic M. How to report statistics in medicine. Philadelphia: American College of Physicians, 1997: 105 – 106.
14 Lang TA, Secic M. How to report statistics in medicine. Philadelphia: American College of Physicians, 1997.
15 Glossary of prosthodontic terms, 8th ed. J Prosthet Dent 2005;94:1 – 81.

M

1 Encarta World English Dictionary [North American Edition]. ©2006. http://encarta.msn.com/dictionary/magnet.html. 2006 June 30.
2 Encarta Encyclopedia English [North American Edition]. ©2006. http://encarta.msn.com/encyclopedia/Magnetism.html. 2006 June 30.
3 Staubli PE, Bagley D. Attachments & implants reference manual, 2nd ed. San Mateo: Attachments International, Inc., 2002.
4 Merriam-Webster's Collegiate Dictionary, 11th ed. Springfield: Merriam-Webster, Inc., 2006. Malpractice litigation; 681, 705.
5 Meijer HJ, Raghoebar GM, Visser A. Mandibular fracture caused by peri-implant bone loss: report of a case. J Periodontol 2003;74(7):1067 – 70.
6 Raghoebar GM, Stellingsma K, Batenburg RH, Vissink A. Etiology and management of mandibular fractures associated with endosteal implants in the atrophic mandible. Oral Surg Oral Med Oral Pathol Oral Radiol Endod 2000;89(5):553 – 9.
7 Pikos MA. Block autografts for localized ridge augmentation: part I. The posterior maxilla. Implant Dent 1999; 8(3):279 – 85.
8 Von Arx T, Hafliger J, Chappuis V. Neurosensory disturbances following bone harvesting in the symphysis: a prospective clinical study. Clin Oral Implants Res 2005; 16(4):432 – 9.

References

9 Canabarro Sde A, Shinkai RS. Medial mandibular flexure and maximum occlusal force in dentate adults. Int J Prosthodont 2006;19:177–182.

10 Zwemer TJ. Boucher's clinical dental terminology, 4th ed. St. Louis: CV Mosby Co., Inc. 1993.

11 Glossary of prosthodontic terms, 8th ed. J Prosthet Dent 2005;94:1–81.

12 Posselt U. Studies in the mobility of the human mandible. Acta Odont Scandinav 1952;10(10):1–160.

13 Sharry JJ. Complete denture prosthodontics, 2nd ed. New York: McGraw-Hill Book Co., Inc., 1962.

14 Itoiz ME, Carranza FA. The gingiva. In: Newman MG, Takei HH, Carranza FA (eds). Carranza's clinical periodontology, 9th ed. Philadelphia: WB Saunders Co., 2002:16–35.

15 Grant DA, Stern IB, Listgarten MA. Periodontics in the tradition of Gottlieb and Orban. 6th ed. St Louis: CV Mosby Co., Inc. 1988.

16 Glossary of prosthodontic terms, 8th ed. J Prosthet Dent 2005;94:29.

17 Jalbout Z, Tabourian G. Glossary of implant dentistry. New Jersey: ICOI and New York University, 2004.

18 Merriam-Webster's Collegiate Dictionary, 11th ed. Springfield: Merriam-Webster, Inc., 2006. Mastication; 764.

19 The anatomical basis of clinical practice. In: Standring S (ed). Gray's anatomy, 39th ed. Toronto: Churchill Livingstone, 2005.

20 Boyne PJ, James RA. Grafting of the maxillary sinus floor with autogenous marrow and bone. J Oral Surg 1980; 38(8):613–6.

21 Tatum H Jr. Maxillary and sinus implant reconstructions. Dent Clin North Am 1986;30(2):207–29.

22 Summers RB. A new concept in maxillary implant surgery: the osteotome technique. Compendium 1994;15(2):152; 154–6; 158; 162.

23 Schwartz-Arad D, Herzberg R, Dolev E. The prevalence of surgical complications of the sinus graft procedure and their impact on implant survival. J Periodontol 2004; 75(4):511–6.

24 Barone A, Santini S, Sbordone L, Crespi R, Covani U. A clinical study of the outcomes and complications associated with maxillary sinus augmentation. Int J Oral Maxillofac Implants 2006;21(1):81–5.

25 Daskalogiannakis J. Glossary of orthodontic terms. Berlin: Quintessence Publishing Co., Inc., 2000:273.

26 Glossary of prosthodontic terms, 8th ed. J Prosthet Dent 2005;94:51.

27 McGivney GP, Castleberry DJ. McCracken's removable partial prosthodontics, 8th ed. St. Louis: CV Mosby Co., Inc. 1989.

28 Feine JS, Carlsson GE, Awad MA, Chehade A, Duncan WJ, Gizani S, et al. The McGill consensus statement on overdentures. Int J Prosthodont 2002;15(4):413–414.

29 Lang TA, Secic M. How to report statistics in medicine. Philadelphia: American College of Physicians, 1997.

30 Williams DF (ed). Definitions in biomaterials. Amsterdam: Elsevier, 1987.

31 The anatomical basis of clinical practice. In: Standring S (ed). Gray's anatomy, 39th ed. Toronto: Churchill Livingstone, 2005.

32 Kemp CK, Hows J, Donaldson C. Bone marrow-derived mesenchymal stem cells. Leuk Lymphoma 2005;46(11): 1531–1544.

33 Goldstein AS. Virginia Polytechnic Institute & State University. Tissue Engineering Laboratory. ©2004. http://www.tissue.che.vt.edu/home_frame.htm. 2006 September 20.

34 Encarta World English Dictionary [North American Edition]. ©2006. http://encarta.msn.com/dictionary/meso.html. 2006 June 30.

35 About, Inc. About.com. ©2006. http://composite.about.com/library/glossary/m/bldef-m3374.htm. 2006 October 23.

36 Glossary of prosthodontic terms, 8th ed. J Prosthet Dent 2005;94:52.

37 Hurley LA, Stinchfield FE, Bassett AL, Lyon WH. The role of soft tissues in osteogenesis. An experimental study of canine spine fusions. J Bone Joint Surg Am 1959;41-A: 1243–54.

38 Murray G, Holden R, Roschlau W. Experimental and clinical study of new growth of bone in a cavity. Am J Surg 1957; 93(3):385–7.

39 Boyne PJ. Regeneration of alveolar bone beneath cellulose acetate filter implants. J Dent Res 1964;43:827.

40 Gottlow J, Nyman S, Karring T, Lindhe J. New attachment formation as the result of controlled tissue regeneration. J Clin Periodontol 1984;11(8):494–503.

41 Nyman S, Gottlow J, Karring T, Lindhe J. The regenerative potential of the periodontal ligament. An experimental study in the monkey. J Clin Periodontol 1982;9(3):257–65.

42 Frost H. Vital biomechanics: proposed general concepts for skeletal adaptations to mechanical usage. Calcif Tissue Int 1988;42:145.

43 Morgan M, James D. Force and moment distributions among osseointegrated dental implants. J Biomech 1995; 28:1103–1109.

44 Zwemer TJ. Boucher's clinical dental terminology, 4th ed. St. Louis: CV Mosby Co., Inc. 1993:75.

45 Garg AK, Mugnolo GM, Sasken H. Maxillary antral mucocele and its relevance for maxillary sinus augmentation grafting: a case report. Int J Oral Maxillofac Implants 2000;15: 287–290.

46 Wennström JL, Pini Prato GP. Mucogingival therapy – periodontal plastic surgery. In: Lindhe J, Karring T, Lang NP (eds). Clinical periodontology and implant dentistry, 4th ed. Oxford: Blackwell Publishing Ltd., 2003:576–649.

47 Glossary of periodontal terms, 4th ed. Chicago: AAP, 2001.

48 Glossary of prosthodontic terms, 8th ed. J Prosthet Dent 2005;94(1):53.

49 Bernard GW, Carranza FA, Jovanovic SA. Biologic aspects of dental implants. In: Newman MG, Takei HH, Carranza FA (eds). Carranza's clinical periodontology, 9th ed. Philadelphia: WB Saunders Co., 2002:882–888.

50 Misch CE. Dental Implant prosthetics. St.Louis: Elsevier Mosby, 2005:75, Fig 6-10.

51 Brånemark PI, Zarb GA, Albrektsson T. Tissue-integrated prostheses: osseointegration in clinical dentistry. Chicago: Quintessence Publishing Co., Inc., 1985.

52 Berman CL. Complications. Dent Clin North Am 1989; 33(4):635–637.

53 McClarence E. Close to the edge. Brånemark and the development of osseointegration. New Malden, London: Quintessence Publishing Co., Ltd., 2003.

54 Lang TA, Secic M. How to report statistics in medicine. Philadelphia: American College of Physicians, 1997: 105–106.

N

1. Beumer J, Curtis TA, Firtell DN. Maxillofacial rehabilitation. St. Louis: CV Mosby Co., Inc. 1979.
2. The anatomical basis of clinical practice. In: Standring S (ed). Gray's anatomy, 39th ed. Toronto: Churchill Livingstone, 2005.
3. Sheets C, Earthman J. Tooth intrusion and reversal in implant-assisted prosthesis: evidence of and a hypothesis for the occurrence. J Prosthet Dent 1993;70:513–520.
4. Peleg M, Mazor Z, Chaushu G, Garg AK. Lateralization of the inferior alveolar nerve with simultaneous implant placement: a modified technique. Int J Oral Maxillofac Implants 2002;17(1):101–6.
5. Gregg JM. Neuropathic complications of mandibular implant surgery: review and case presentations. Ann R Australas Coll Dent Surg 2000;15:176–80.
6. Garg AK, Morales MJ. Lateralization of the inferior alveolar nerve with simultaneous implant placement: surgical techniques. Pract Periodontics Aesthet Dent 1998;10(9):1197–204; 1206.
7. Hirsch JM, Brånemark PI. Fixture stability and nerve function after transposition and lateralization of the inferior alveolar nerve and fixture installation. J Oral Maxillofac Surg 1995;33(5):276–81.
8. American Academy of Periodontology. Surgical therapy. In: Hallmon WW, Carranza FA Jr, Drisko CL, Rapley JW, Robinson P (eds). Periodontal literature reviews – a summary of current knowledge. Chicago: AAP, 1996:145–203.
9. Gilboe DB, Teteruck WR. Fundamentals of extracoronal tooth preparation. Part I. Retention and resistance form. J Prosthet Dent 1974;32(6):651–6.
10. Aboyoussef H, Weiner S, Ehrenberg D. Effect of an antirotation resistance form on screw loosening for single implant-supported crowns. J Prosthet Dent 2000;83(4):450–5.
11. Proussaefs P, Campagni W, Bernal G, Goodacre C, Kim J. The effectiveness of auxiliary features on a tooth preparation with inadequate resistance form. J Prosthet Dent 2004;91(1):33–41.
12. Listgarten MA, Buser D, Steinemann SG, Donath K, Lang NP, Weber HP. Light and transmission electron microscopy of the intact interfaces between non-submerged titanium-coated epoxy resin implants and bone or gingiva. J Dent Res 1992;71(2):364–71. Erratum in: J Dent Res 1992;71(5):1267.
13. Buser D, Weber HP, Lang NP. Tissue integration of non-submerged implants. 1-year results of a prospective study with 100 ITI hollow-cylinder and hollow-screw implants. Clin Oral Implants Res 1990;1(1):33–40.
14. Cochran DL, Mahn DH. Dental Implants and Regeneration Part I. Overview and Biological Considerations. In: Clark's Clinical Dentistry Volume 5. Philadelphia: J.B. Lippincott Company 1993: Ch 59:3, Fig 3.
15. Glossary of prosthodontic terms, 8th ed. J Prosthet Dent 2005;94:1–81.
16. Lang TA, Secic M. How to report statistics in medicine. Philadelphia: American College of Physicians, 1997.

O

1. Jalbout Z, Tabourian G. Glossary of implant dentistry. New Jersey: ICOI and New York University, 2004.
2. Glossary of prosthodontic terms, 8th ed. J Prosthet Dent 2005;94:1–81.
3. Zwemer TJ. Boucher's clinical dental terminology, 4th ed. St. Louis: CV Mosby Co., Inc. 1993.
4. Beumer J, Curtis TA, Firtell DN. Maxillofacial rehabilitation, St. Louis: CV Mosby Co., Inc. 1979.
5. Daskalogiannakis J. Glossary of orthodontic terms. Berlin: Quintessence Publishing Co., Inc., 2000.
6. Cehreli MC, Akca K, Iplikcioglu H. Force transmission of one- and two-piece Morse-taper oral implants: a nonlinear finite element analysis. Clin Oral Impl Res 2005;15:481–489.
7. Hermann JS, Buser D, Schenk RK, Schoolfield JD, Cochran DL. Biologic width around one- and two-piece titanium implants. A histometric evaluation of unloaded nonsubmerged and submerged implants in the canine mandible. Clin Oral Impl Res 2001;12:559–571.
8. Glossary of periodontal terms, 4th ed. Chicago: AAP, 2001.
9. Slade GD, Spencer AJ. Development and evaluation of the oral health impact profile. Community Dent Health 1994;11:3–11.
10. Inglehart MR, Bagramian RA. Oral health-related quality of life. Chicago: Quintessence Publishing Co., Inc., 2002.
11. Brånemark PI, Zarb GA, Albrektsson T. Tissue-integrated prostheses: osseointegration in clinical dentistry. Chicago: Quintessence Publishing Co., Inc., 1985.
12. Schenk RK, Hjørting-Hansen E, Buser D. Bone integration of implants. Forum Implantologicum 2006;2:14–23.
13. Jacobs R, van Steenberghe D. From osseoperception to implant-mediated sensory-motor interactions and related clinical implications. J Oral Rehab 2006; 33(4)282–92.
14. Theill LE, Boyle WJ, Penninger JM. RANK-L and RANK: T-cells, bone loss, and mammalian evolution. Ann Rev Immunol 2002;20:795-823, Fig 2.
15. Buser D, Dahlin C, Schenk R.K. Guided bone regeneration in implant dentistry. Chicago: Quintessence Publishing Co., Inc. 1994:52, Fig 3-2.
16. Schroeder A, Sutter F, Krekeler G. Oral implantology. New York: Thieme Verlag Stuttgart, 1991.
17. Buser D, Dahlin C, Schenk, RK. Guided bone regeneration in implant dentistry. Chicago: Quintessence Publishing Co., Inc., 1994:34, Fig 2-1.
18. Simonet WS, Lacey DL, Dunstan CR, Kelley M, Chang MS, Luthy R, et al. Osteoprotegerin: a novel secreted protein involved in the regulation of bone density. Cell 1997;89:309–319.
19. Rosen PS, Summers R, Mellado JR, Salkin LM, Shanaman RH, Marks MH, Fugazzotto PA. The bone-added osteotome sinus floor elevation technique: multicenter retrospective report of consecutively treated patients. Int J Oral Maxillofac Implants 1999;14(6):853–8.
20. Summers RB. A new concept in maxillary implant surgery: the osteotome technique. Compendium 1994;15(2):152; 154–6; 158; 162.
21. ASTM Dictionary of Engineering Science and Technology, 9th ed. West Conshohocken: ASTM, 2000. Oxide surfaces; 562.

References

P

[1] Tarnow DP, Magner AW, Fletcher P. The effect of the distance from the contact point to the crest of bone on the presence or absence of the interproximal dental papilla. J Periodontol 1992;63(12):995–6.

[2] Tarnow DP, Cho SC, Wallace SS. The effect of inter-implant distance on the height of inter-implant bone crest. J Periodontol 2000;71(4):546–9.

[3] Choquet V, Hermans M, Adriaenssens P, Daelemans P, Tarnow DP, Malevez C. Clinical and radiographic evaluation of the papilla level adjacent to single-tooth dental implants. A retrospective study in the maxillary anterior region. J Periodontol 2001;72(10):1364–71.

[4] Tarnow D, Elian N, Fletcher P, Froum S, Magner A, Cho SC et al. Vertical distance from the crest of bone to the height of the interproximal papilla between adjacent implants. J Periodontol 2003;74(12):1785–8.

[5] Glossary of prosthodontic terms, 8th ed. J Prosthet Dent 2005;94:1–81.

[6] Xu H, Shimizu Y, Asai S, Ooya K. Experimental sinus grafting with the use of deproteinized bone particles of different sizes. Clin Oral Implants Res 2003;14(5):548–55.

[7] Pallesen L, Schou S, Aaboe M, Hjorting-Hansen E, Nattestad A, Melsen F. Influence of particle size of autogenous bone grafts on the early stages of bone regeneration: a histologic and stereologic study in rabbit calvarium. Int J Oral Maxillofac Implants 2002;17(4):498–506.

[8] Shapoff CA, Bowers GM, Levy B, Mellonig JT, Yukna RA. The effect of particle size on the osteogenic activity of composite grafts of allogeneic freeze-dried bone and autogenous marrow. J Periodontol 1980;51(11):625–30.

[9] Fitzpatrick R, Davey C, Buxton MJ, Jones DR. Evaluating patient-based outcome measures for use in clinical trials. Health Technol Assessment 1998;2(14).

[10] Quality Assurance Project. Methods and tools. http://www.qaproject.org/methods/resglossary.html. 2006 June 30.

[11] Glossary of periodontal terms, 4th ed. Chicago: AAP, 2001.

[12] Ito T, Johnson JD. Color atlas of periodontal surgery. Barcelona: Espax, SA Publicaciones Medicas, 1994: Ch 10, p 197, Fig 10-71.

[13] Merck Source. Resource Library. ©2007. http://www.mercksource.com/pp/us/cns/cns_search_results.jsp. 2007 May 23.

[14] Albrektsson T, Brånemark PI, Hansson HA, Lindstrom J. Osseointegrated titanium implants. Requirements for ensuring a long-lasting, direct bone-to-implant anchorage in man. Acta Orthop Scand 1981;52(2):155–70.

[15] Brånemark PI, Tolman DE. Osseointegration in craniofacial reconstruction, Chicago: Quintessence Publishing Co., Inc., 1998:69.

[16] Grant DA, Stern IB, Listgarten MA. Periodontics in the tradition of Gottlieb and Orban. 6th ed. St Louis: CV Mosby Co., Inc. 1988.

[17] Sarment DP, Peshman B. Manual of dental implants. Hudson, Ohio: Lexi-Comp, Inc., 2004.

[18] Miller PD Jr. A classification of marginal tissue recession. Int J Periodontics Restorative Dent 1985;5(2):8–13.

[19] Falkner M, Woolfaardt J, Chan A. Measuring abutment/implant joint integrity with the Periotest instrument. Int J Oral Maxillofac Implants 1999;14:681–688, Fig 1.

[20] Zwemer TJ. Boucher's clinical dental terminology, 4th ed. St. Louis: CV Mosby Co., Inc. 1993.

[21] Lodish H., Berk H.A., Zipursky L.S., Matsudaira P, Baltimore D, Darnell J. Molecular Cell Biology, 4th ed. New York: W. H. Freeman and Company, 2000: Ch 7, p 209, Fig 7.1.

[22] Berman I. Color atlas of basic histology, 2nd ed. Stamford: Appleton & Lange, 1998: Ch 8, p 87, Fig 8-10.

[23] Bhanot S, Alex JC. Current applications of platelet gels in facial plastic surgery. Facial Plast Surg 2002;18(1): 27–33.

[24] Anitua E, Sanchez M, Nurden AT, Nurden P, Orive G, Andia I. New insights into and novel applications for platelet-rich fibrin therapies. Trends Biotechnol 2006; 24(5): 227–234.

[25] Marx RE, Carlson ER, Eichstaedt RM, Schimmele SR, Strauss JE, Georgeff KR. Platelet-rich plasma: growth factor enhancement for bone grafts. Oral Surg Oral Med Oral Pathol Oral Radiol Endod 1998;85(6):638–46.

[26] Jalbout Z, Tabourian G. Glossary of implant dentistry. New Jersey: ICOI and New York University, 2004.

[27] Yanase RT, Preston JD. Nomenclature for implant dentistry. In: Fonseca R, Davis WH (eds). Reconstructive and prepros-thetic oral and maxillofacial surgery. 2nd ed. Philadelphia: WB Saunders Co., 1995:233.

[28] Zarb GA, Bergman B, Clayton JA, MacKay, HF. Prosthodontic treatment for partially edentulous patients. St. Louis: CV Mosby Co., Inc. 1978:379.

[29] Encarta World English Dictionary [North American Edition]. ©2006. http://encarta.msn.com/dictionary_/prefabricated.html. 2006 June 30.

[30] Glossary of prosthodontic terms, 8th ed. J Prosthet Dent 2005;94:63.

[31] U.S. Food and Drug Administration, Center for Devices and Radiological Heath. http://www.fda.gov/cdrh/devadvice/314.html. 2004 January 14.

[32] Lang TA, Secic M. How to report statistics in medicine. Philadelphia: American College of Physicians, 1997.

[33] Glossary of prosthodontic terms, 8th ed. J Pros Dent 2005;84:73.

[34] Raghavendra S, Wood M, Taylor T. Early wound healing around endosseous implants: a review of the literature. Int J Oral Maxillofac Implants 2005;20:425–431.

[35] Newman MG, Takei H, Carranza FA, Klokkevold PR (eds). Carranza's clinical periodontology, 10th ed. Philadelphia: WB Saunders Company, 2006: Ch 35, p 552, Fig 35-18.

[36] Wennerberg A, Albrektsson T. Suggested guidelines for the topographical evaluation of implant surfaces. Int J Oral Maxillofac Implants 2000;15:331–344.

[37] The American Heritage Stedman's Medical Dictionary, 2nd ed. ©2004. http://medical-dictionary.thefreedictionary.com/proprioception. 2006 June 30.

[38] Jacobs R, van Steenberghe D. From osseoperception to implant-mediated sensory-motor interactions and related clinical implications. J Oral Rehabil 2006;33:282–292.

[39] Lundborg G. The role of osseointegration in joint replacement - hand surgical aspects. In: Albrektsson T, Zarb G (eds). The Brånemark osseointegrated implant. Chicago: Quintessence Publishing Co., Inc., 1989:245.

[40] Yanase RT, Preston JD. Nomenclature for implant dentistry. In: Fonseca R, Davis WH (eds). Reconstructive and prepros-thetic oral and maxillofacial surgery. 2nd ed. Philadelphia: WB Saunders Co., 1995:235–237.

[41] Merck Source. Resource Library. ©2006. http://www.mercksource.com/pp/us/cns/cns_search_results.jsp. 2007 May 8.

[42] IFFGD. Glossary of Terms. ©2006. http://iffgd.org/GIDisorders/glossary.html. 2006 June 30.

[43] Balshi TJ. A provisional fixed prosthesis supported by osseointegrated titanium fixture. In: The conversion prosthesis; Exerpta Medica. International Congress on Tissue Integration in Oral and Maxillofacial Reconstruction. Brussels, Belgium, May 1985.

[44] Vrielinck L, Politis C, Schepers S, Pauwels M, Naert I. Image-based planning and clinical validation of zygoma and pterygoid implant placement in patients with severe bone atrophy using customized drill guides. Preliminary results from a prospective clinical follow-up study. Int J Oral Maxillofac Surg 2003;32(1):7–14.

[45] Graves SL. The pterygoid plate implant: a solution for restoring the posterior maxilla. Int J Periodontics Restorative Dent 1994;14(6):512–23.

Q

____

R

[1] Roberts R. Ramus frame mandibular implant. Clark's Clin Dent 1987;5:1–11.

[2] Turner HF. Ramus frame implant technique. J Am Dent Asso 1990;121(3):418–420.

[3] Staubli PE, Bagley D. Attachments & implants reference manual, 2nd ed. San Mateo: Attachments International, Inc., 2002.

[4] Lang TA, Secic M. How to report statistics in medicine. Philadelphia: American College of Physicians, 1997.

[5] Encarta World English Dictionary [North American Edition]. ©2006. http://encarta.msn.com/dictionary_/ratchet.html. 2006 June 15.

[6] The American Academy of Periodontology. Periodontal literature reviews. A summary of current knowledge. Chicago: AAP, 1996.

[7] Khosla S. Minireview. The OPG/RANKL/RANK system. Endocrinology 2001;142(12):5050–5055.

[8] Zwemer TJ. Boucher's clinical dental terminology, 4th ed. St. Louis: CV Mosby Co., Inc. 1993.

[9] Glossary of prosthodontic terms, 8th ed. J Prosthet Dent 2005;94:1–81.

[10] Frost HM. The regional acceleratory phenomenon: a review. Henry Ford Hosp Med J 1983;31(1):3–9.

[11] Yanase RT, Preston JD. Nomenclature for implant dentistry. In: Fonseca R, Davis WH (eds). Reconstructive and preprosthetic oral and maxillofacial surgery, 2nd ed. Philadelphia: WB Saunders Co., 1995:233.

[12] Araujo MG, Lindhe J. Dimensional ridge alterations following tooth extraction. An experimental study in the dog. J Clin Periodontol 2005;32(2):212–8.

[13] Merriam-Webster's Collegiate Dictionary, 11th ed. Springfield: Merriam-Webster, Inc., 2006. Resin; 1060.

[14] Meredith N, Alleyne D, Cawley P. Quantitative determination of the stability of the implant-tissue interface using resonance frequency analysis. Clin Oral Implants Res 1996; 7:261–267, p 263, Fig 2.

[15] Andreasen JO, Andreasen FM. Textbook and color atlas of traumatic injuries, 3rd ed. Copenhagen: Munksgaard, Copenhagen 1994:395, Fig 10-16.

[16] Yanase RT, Preston JD. Nomenclature for implant dentistry. In: Fonseca R, Davis WH (eds). Reconstructive and preprosthetic oral and maxillofacial surgery, 2nd ed. Philadelphia: WB Saunders Co., 1995:232.

[17] Daskalogiannakis J. Glossary of Orthodontic Terms. Berlin: Quintessence Publishing Co., Inc., 2000.

[18] Merriam-Webster's Collegiate Dictionary, 11th ed. Springfield: Merriam-Webster, Inc., 2006. Retention; 1064.

[19] Yanase RT, Preston JD. Nomenclature for implant dentistry. In: Fonseca R, Davis WH (eds). Reconstructive and preprosthetic oral and maxillofacial surgery, 2nd ed. Philadelphia: WB Saunders Co., 1995:234.

[20] Merriam-Webster's Collegiate Dictionary, 11th ed. Springfield: Merriam-Webster, Inc., 2006. Retraction cord; 277.

[21] Jalbout Z, Tabourian G. Glossary of implant dentistry. New Jersey: ICOI and New York University, 2004.

[22] Sullivan D, Sherwood R, Collinis T, Krogh P. The reverse-torque test: a clinical report. Int J Oral Maxillofac Implants 1996;11:179–185.

[23] Stein RS. Mutual protective complex of dental restorations. In: Laney WR, Gibilisco JA. Diagnosis and Treatment in Prosthodontics. Philadelphia: Lea and Febiger, 1983:322.

[24] Newman MG, Takei HH, Carranza FA. Clinical periodontology. Philadelphia: WB Saunders Co., 2002.

[25] Lindhe J, Karring T, Lang NP (eds.). Clinical periodontology and implant dentistry, 4th ed. Oxford: Blackwell Publishing Ltd., 2003.

[26] Glossary of prosthodontic terms, 8th ed. J Prosthet Dent 2005;94(1):70.

[27] Yanase RT, Preston JD. Considerations for screw/cylinder prosthetic components. In: Fonseca R, Davis WH, (eds). Reconstructive preprosthetic oral and maxillofacial surgery, 2nd ed. Philadelphia: WB Saunders Co., 1995:227.

[28] Albrektsson T, Wennerberg A. Oral implant surfaces: review focusing on topographic and chemical responses to them. Int J Prosthodont 2004;17:536–543.

[29] Wennerberg A, Albrektsson T. Suggested guidelines for the topographical evaluation of implant surfaces. Int J Oral Maxillofac Implants 2000;15:331–344.

S

[1] Wei G, Jin Q, Giannobile WV, Ma PX. Nano-fibrous scaffold for controlled delivery of recombinant human PDGF-BB. J Control Release 2006;112(1):103–110, Fig 2.

[2] Illustrated Stedman's medical dictionary, 24th ed. Baltimore: Williams & Wilkins, 1982. Screw; 1267.

[3] Encarta World English Dictionary [North American Edition]. ©2006. http://encarta.msn.com/dictionary_/screw.html. 2006 June 15.

[4] Jalbout Z, Tabourian G. Glossary of implant dentistry. New Jersey: ICOI and New York University, 2004.

[5] Yanase RT, Preston JD. Nomenclature for implant dentistry. In: Fonseca R, Davis WH (eds). Reconstructive and preprosthetic oral and maxillofacial surgery, 2nd ed. Philadelphia: WB Saunders Co., 1995:235.

References

6 Yanase RT, Preston JD. Nomenclature for implant dentistry. In: Fonseca R, Davis WH (eds). Reconstructive and preprosthetic oral and maxillofacial surgery, 2nd ed. Philadelphia: WB Saunders Co., 1995:230 – 231.

7 Raghavendra S, Wood M, Taylor T. Early wound healing around endosseous implants: a review of the literature. Int J Oral Maxillofac Implants 2005;20:425 – 431.

8 Rangert B, Jemt T, Jorneus L. Forces and moments on Brånemark implants. Int J Oral Maxillofac Implants 1989;4: 241 – 247, Fig 3.

9 Staubli PE, Bagley D. Attachments & implants reference manual. 2nd ed. San Mateo: Attachments International, Inc., 2002:166.

10 Lindhe J, Karring T, Lang NP (eds.). Clinical periodontology and implant dentistry, 4th ed. Oxford: Blackwell Publishing Ltd., 2003: Ch 1, p 42, Fig 1-91.

11 Lang TA, Secic M. How to report statistics in medicine. Philadelphia: American College of Physicians, 1997.

12 Merriam-Webster's Collegiate Dictionary, 11th ed. Springfield: Merriam-Webster, Inc., 2006. Silicone; 1160.

13 Zwemer TJ. Boucher's clinical dental terminology, 4th ed. St Louis: CV Mosby Co., Inc. 1993.

14 Lang TA, Secic M. How to report statistics in medicine. Philadelphia: American College of Physicians, 1997: 105 – 106.

15 Merriam-Webster's Collegiate Dictionary, 11th ed. Springfield: Merriam-Webster, Inc., 2006. Simulation; 1162.

16 Glossary of prosthodontic terms, 8th ed. J Prosthet Dent 2005;84:72.

17 Jensen OT, Shulman LB, Block MS, Iacono VJ. Report of the sinus consensus conference of 1996. Int J Oral Maxillofac Implants 1998;13:11 – 45 (Special Supplement).

18 Skalak R. Biomechanical considerations in osseointegrated prostheses. J Prosthet Dent 1983;49:843 – 848.

19 Skalak R. Aspects of biomechanical considerations. In: Brånemark PI, Zarb GA, Albrektsson T (eds). Tissue-Integrated Prostheses: Osseointegration in Clinical Dentistry. Chicago: Quintessence Publishing Co., Inc., 1985:121 – 122, Fig 5-2, 5-3, 5-4a, 5-4b.

20 Taylor TD. Clinical maxillofacial prosthetics. Chicago: Quintessence Publishing Co., Inc., 2000.

21 Cochran D, Simpson J, Weber H, Buser D. Attachment and growth of periodontal cells on smooth and rough titanium. Int J Oral Maxillofac Implants 1994;9:291, Fig 3a, 3b.

22 Glossary of prosthodontic terms, 8th ed. J Prosthet Dent 2005;94:1 – 81.

23 Merriam-Webster's Collegiate Dictionary, 11th ed. Springfield: Merriam-Webster, Inc., 2006. Smile; 1177.

24 Frush JP, Fisher RD. Introduction to dentogenic restoration. J Prosthet Dent 1955;5:586 – 595.

25 Frush JP, Fisher RD. How dentogenic restorations interpret the personality factor. J Prosthet Dent 1956;6:441 – 449.

26 Aiba N. Dentscape - functional esthetic. Quintessence J Dent Technol 2006;29:89.

27 Quintessence of Dental Technology. Chicago: Quintessence Publishing Co., Inc., 2006:119, Fig 21.

28 Watzek G. Endosseous implants: scientific and clinical aspects. Chicago: Quintessence Publishing Co., Inc., 1996: 392, Fig 11-39a.

29 Laney WR, Gibilisco JA. Diagnosis and treatment in prosthodontics. Philadelphia: Lea and Febiger, 1983:346 – 357.

30 Ingraham JL, Ingraham CA. Introduction to microbiology, 2nd ed. Pacific Grove: Brooks/Cole, 2000: Ch 4, p 99, Fig 4.11b.

31 Merriam-Webster's Collegiate Dictionary, 11th ed. Springfield: Merriam-Webster, Inc., 2006. Splinting; 1205.

32 Merriam-Webster's Collegiate Dictionary, 11th ed. Springfield: Merriam-Webster, Inc., 2006. Stability; 1213.

33 Brånemark PI, Zarb GA, Albrektsson T. Tissue-integrated prostheses-osseointegration in clinical dentistry. Chicago: Quintessence Publishing Co., Inc., 1985:236.

34 St. Jude's Children's Research Hospital. Medical Terminology and Drug Database. ©2006. http://www.stjude.org/glossary. 2006 June 30.

35 Von Arx T, Cochran D, Hermann J, Schenk R, Higginbottom F, Buser D. Lateral ridge augmentation and implant placement: an experimental study evaluating implant osseointegration in different augmentation materials in the canine mandible. Int J Oral Maxillofac Implants 2001;16:343 – 354.

36 Langer B, Langer L. Subepithelial connective tissue graft technique for root coverage. J Periodontol 1985;56(12): 715 – 20.

37 The anatomical basis of clinical practice. In: Standring S (ed). Gray's anatomy, 39th ed. Toronto: Churchill Livingstone, 2005.

38 Cochran DL, Mahn DH. Dental Implants and Regeneration Part I. Overview and Biological Considerations. In: Clark's Clinical Dentistry Volume 5. Philadelphia: J.B. Lippincott Company 1993: Ch 59:3, Fig 2.

39 Fiorellini JP, Engebretson SP, Donath K, Weber HP. Guided bone regeneration utilizing expanded polytetrafluoroethylene membranes in combination with submerged and nonsubmerged dental implants in beagle dogs. J Periodontol 1998:69:528 – 535.

40 Gershkoff A, Goldberg NI. The implant lower denture. Dent Digest 1949;55:490 – 494.

41 Sato N. Periodontal surgery - a clinical atlas. Chicago: Quintessence Publishing Co., Inc., 2000:25, Fig 1-8.

42 Taylor TD, Laney WR. Dental implants: are they for me? Chicago: Quintessence Publishing Co., Inc., 1993.

43 The American Heritage Stedman's Medical Dictionary, 2nd ed. ©2004. http://medical-dictionary.thefreedictionary.com/ suppuration. 2006 June 30.

44 Willams DF, Roaf F. Implants in surgery. London: WB Saunders Co., Ltd., 1973.

45 Casap N, Tarazi E, Wexler A, Sonnenfeld U, Lustmann J. Intraoperative computerized navigation for flapless implant surgery and immediate loading in the edentulous mandible. Int J Oral Maxillofac Implants 2005;20:92 – 98.

46 Wennerberg A, Albrektsson T. Suggested guidelines for the topographical evaluation of implant surfaces. Int J Oral Maxillofac Implants 2000;15:331 – 344.

T

1 Yanase RT, Preston JD. Nomenclature for implant dentistry. In: Fonseca R, Davis WH (eds). Reconstructive and preprosthetic oral and maxillofacial surgery, 2nd ed. Philadelphia: WB Saunders Co., 1995:232.

2 Brånemark PI, Zarb GA, Albrektsson T. Tissue-integrated prostheses: osseointegration in clinical dentistry. Chicago: Quintessence Publishing Co., Inc., 1985.

[3] Berman CL. Complications. Dent Clin North Am 1989;33(4): 635–637.

[4] McClarence E. Close to the edge. Brånemark and the development of osseointegration. New Malden, London: Quintessence Publishing Co., Ltd., 2003.

[5] Babbush CA. Kirsch A. Mentag PJ. Hill B. Intramobile cylinder (IMZ) two-stage osteointegrated implant system with the intramobile element (IME): part I. Its rationale and procedure for use. Int J Oral Maxillofac Implants 1987;2(4): 203–216.

[6] Shillingburg HT, Hobo S, Whitsett LD, Jacobi R, Brackett SE. Fundamentals of fixed prosthodontics, 3rd ed. Chicago: Quintessence Publishing Co., Inc., 1997.

[7] Brewer AA, Morrow RM. Overdentures, 2nd ed. St. Louis: CV Mosby Co., Inc. 1980:209–10.

[8] Weischer T, Schettler D, Mohr C. Implant-supported telescopic restorations in maxillofacial prosthetics. Int J Prosthodont 1997;10(3):287–92.

[9] Rokni SR. Combination acid-etched and coping-superstructure fixed partial prosthesis. Quintessence Int 1996;27(3): 189–92.

[10] Gray H. Gray's anatomy, 15th ed. New York: Barnes and Noble, Inc., 1995.

[11] Boucher CO. Swenson's complete dentures, 6th ed. St. Louis: CV Mosby Co., Inc. 1970.

[12] Gray H. Gray's anatomy, 15th ed. New York: Barnes and Noble, Inc., 1995:203–204.

[13] Jalbout Z, Tabourian G. Glossary of implant dentistry. New Jersey: ICOI and New York University, 2004.

[14] The anatomical basis of clinical practice. In: Standring S (ed). Gray's anatomy, 39th ed. Toronto: Churchill Livingstone, 2005.

[15] Mazock JB, Schow SR, Triplett RG. Proximal tibia bone harvest: review of technique, complications, and use in maxillofacial surgery. Int J Oral Maxillofac Implants 2004;19(4): 586–93.

[16] Lytle RB. The management of abused oral tissues in complete denture construction. J Prosthet Dent 1957;7:27–42.

[17] Chase WW. Tissue conditioning utilizing dynamic adaptive stress. J Prosthet Dent 1961;11:804–815.

[18] McCarthy JA, Moser JB. Mechanical properties of tissue conditioners. Part I. Theoretical considerations, behavioral characteristics, and tensile properties. Part II. Creep characteristics. J Prosthet Dent 1978;40:89-97;334–342.

[19] Laney WR, Gibilisco JA. Diagnosis and treatment in prosthodontics. Philadelphia: Lea and Febiger, 1983.

[20] Brånemark PI, Zarb GA, Albrektsson T. Tissue-integrated prostheses: osseointegration in clinical dentistry. Chicago: Quintessence Publishing Co., Inc., 1985:311, Fig 17-52.

[21] Buser D, Dahlin C, Schenk RK. Guided bone regeneration in implant dentistry. Chicago: Quintessence Publishing Co., Inc. 1994:66, Fig 3-15a, 3-15b, 3-15c.

[22] Glossary of prosthodontic terms, 8th ed. J Prosthet Dent 2005;94(1):78.

[23] Gatti C, Chiapasco M. Immediate loading of Brånemark implants: a 24-month follow-up of a comparative prospective pilot study between mandibular overdentures supported by conical transmucosal and standard MK II implants. Clin Imp Dent Rel Res 2002;4(4):190–9.

[24] Hammerle CH, Lang NP. Single-stage surgery combining transmucosal implant placement with guided bone regeneration and bioresorbable materials. Clin Oral Implants Res 2001;12(1):9–18.

[25] Bosker H. The transmandibular implant. Dissertation 1941, University of Utrecht, The Netherlands.

[26] Reuther T, Schuster T, Mende U, Kubler A. Osteoradionecrosis of the jaws as a side effect of radiotherapy of head and neck tumour patients - a report of a thirty-year retrospective review. Int J Oral Maxillofac Surg 2003;32(3):289–95.

[27] Marx RE, Ehler WJ, Tayapongsak P, Pierce LW. Relationship of oxygen dose to angiogenesis induction in irradiated tissue. Am J Surg 1990;160(5):519–24.

[28] Buser D, von Arx T, ten Bruggenkate C, Weingart D. Basic surgical principles with ITI implants. Clin Oral Implants Res 2000;11(1):59–68.

[29] Glossary of prosthodontic terms, 8th ed. J Prosthet Dent 2005;94:1–81.

[30] Zwemer TJ. Boucher's clinical dental terminology, 4th ed. St. Louis: CV Mosby Co., Inc. 1993.

[31] Lang TA, Secic M. How to report statistics in medicine. Philadelphia: American College of Physicians, 1997.

[32] Cehreli MC, Akca K, Iplikcioglu H. Force transmission of one- and two-piece morse-taper oral implants: a nonlinear finite element analysis. Clin Oral Impl Res 2005;15:481–489.

[33] Hermann JS, Buser D, Schenk RK, Schoolfield JD, Cochran DL. Biologic width around one- and two-piece titanium implants. A histometric evaluation of unloaded nonsubmerged and submerged implants in the canine mandible. Clin Oral Impl Res 2001;12:559–571.

U

[1] Lewis S, Beumer J, Hornburg W, Moy P. The "UCLA" abutment. Int J Oral Maxillofac Implants 1988;3(3):183–9.

[2] Lewis SG, Llamas D, Avera S. The UCLA abutment: a four-year review. J Prosthet Dent 1992;67(4):509–15.

[3] Schortinghuis J. Ultrasound stimulation of mandibular bone healing. Thesis. University of Groeningen, The Netherlands, 2004.

V

[1] Merriam-Webster's Collegiate Dictionary, 11th ed. Springfield: Merriam-Webster, Inc., 2006. Valsalva maneuver; 1382.

[2] Lang TA, Secic M. How to report statistics in medicine. Philadelphia: American College of Physicians, 1997.

[3] Zwemer TJ. Boucher's clinical dental terminology, 4th ed. St. Louis: CV Mosby Co., Inc. 1993.

[4] Glossary of prosthodontic terms, 8th ed. J Prosthet Dent 2005;94:1–81.

[5] Jalbout Z, Tabourian G. Glossary of implant dentistry. New Jersey: ICOI and New York University, 2004.

[6] Procera Laboratory Manual. Goteborg: Nobel Biocare AB.

[7] Darley FL. Speech pathology. In: Laney WR, Gibilisco JA (eds). Diagnosis and treatment in prosthodontics. Philadelphia: Lea and Febiger, 1983:346–376.

[8] Silverman MM. The speaking method in measuring vertical dimension. J Prosthet Dent 1953;3:193–199.

[9] Uitterlinden AG, Fang Y, Van Meurs JBJ, Pols HAP, van Leeuwen, JPTM. Genetics and biology of vitamin D receptor polymorphisms. Gene 2004; 338:143–56.

References

10 Andrades PR, Calderon W, Leniz P, Bartel G, Danilla S, Benitez S. Geometric analysis of the V-Y advancement flap and its clinical applications. Plast Reconstr Surg 2005;115(6): 1582 – 90.

W

1 Zwemer TJ. Boucher's clinical dental terminology, 4th ed. St. Louis: CV Mosby Co., Inc. 1993.
2 Glossary of prosthodontic terms, 8th ed. J Prosthet Dent 2005:94:1 – 81.
3 Jalbout Z, Tabourian G. Glossary of implant dentistry. New Jersey: ICOI and New York University, 2004:55.
4 Cranin N. Glossary of implant terms. J Oral Implantol 2003;29:1 – 1.
5 Wolff J. Das Gesetz der Transformation der Knochen. Berlin: A Hirschwald, 1891.
6 Salter R. Textbook of disorders and injuries of the musculoskeletal system. Baltimore: Williams and Wilkens, 1970.
7 Watzek G. Implants in qualitatively compromised bone. Berlin: Quintessence Publishing Co., Inc. 2004:13, Fig 2-1a, 2-1b, 2-1c.

X

——

Y

——

Z

1 Esposito M, Worthington HV, Coulthard P: Interventions for replacing missing teeth: dental implants in zygomatic bone for the rehabilitation of the severely deficient edentulous maxilla (review). Cochrane Database of Systematic Reviews 2005;4;2:1.
2 Boyes-Varley JG, Howes DG, Lownie JF, Blackbeard GA. Surgical modifications to the Brånemark zygomaticus protocol in the treatment of the severely resorbed maxilla: a clinical report. J Oral Maxillofac Implants 2003:18:232 – 237.

Trademark Appendix

A. Titan, Instruments
97 Main Street
Hamburg, NY 14075, USA
Phone (877) 284-8261; (716) 648-9272
Fax (716) 648-9296
www.atitan.com

AccuDental Guided Implant Modeling
Medical Modeling, LLC
17301 West Colfax Avenue, Suite 300
Golden, CO 80401, USA
Phone (888) 273-5344
Fax (303) 273-6463
www.medicalmodeling.com

ACE Surgical Supply Company, Inc.
1034 Pearl Street
Brockton, MA 02301, USA
Phone (800) 441-3100; (508) 588-3100
Fax (800) 583-3150; (508) 583-3140
www.acesurgical.com

Advanced Implant Technologies, Inc.
8920 Wilshire Boulevard, Suite 305
Beverly Hills, CA 90211, USA
Phone (800) 876-4620; (310) 652-9314
Fax (800) 298-2383; (310) 659-1594
www.aitdental.com

Alphadent N.V.
Ceka Center
Noorderlaan 79
2030 Antwerpen, BELGIUM
Phone (32) 3 542 25 27
Fax (32) 3 542 24 30
http://alphadent.ys.be/ceka/en/about/

Aseptico, Inc.
8333 216th Street, SE
Woodinville, WA 98072-1548, USA
Phone (425) 487-3157; (800) 426-5913
Fax (360) 668-8722
www.aseptico.com

AstraTech, Inc.
890 Winter Street, Suite 310
Waltham, MA 02451, USA
Phone (800) 531-3481; (781) 890-6808
Fax (781) 890-6808
www.astratech.com

Atlantis Components, Inc.
25 First Street
Cambridge, MA 02141, USA
Phone (877) 828-5268
Fax (617) 661-9063
www.atlantiscomp.com

Attachments International, Inc.
600 South Amphlett Boulevard
San Mateo, CA 94402-1325, USA
Phone (Ordering) (800) 999-3003
Phone (Technical Support) (650) 340-1426
Fax (650) 340-8423
www.attachments.com

Bicon Dental Implants
501 Arborway
Boston, MA 02130, USA
Phone (800) 882-4266; (617) 524-4443
Fax (800) 882-4266; (617) 524-0096
www.bicon.com

BioHorizons Implant Systems, Inc.
One Perimeter Park South, Suite 230 S
Birmingham, AL 35243, USA
Phone (888) 246-8338; (205) 967-7880
Fax (205) 870-0304
www.biohorizons.com

BioLok International, Inc.
(formerly Minimatic Implant Technology, Inc.)
368 South Military Trail
Deerfield Beach, FL 33442, USA
Phone (800) 789-0830; (954) 698-9998
Fax (954) 698-9925
www.biolok.com

Bredent USA – XPDent Corporation
12145 SW 131 Avenue
Miami, FL 33186, USA
Phone (800) 328-3965; (305) 233-3312
Fax (305) 233-2002
www.xpdent.com

CAMLOG Biotechnologies USA
Granite Woods
Corporate Center, Buildg. 2
350 Granite Street
Braintree, MA 02184, USA
Phone (877) 537-8862
Fax (877) 418 2365
www.camlogimplants.com

CAMLOG Vertriebs GmbH
Maybachstrasse 5
71299 Wimsheim, GERMANY
Phone 49 (0) 7044-9445-0
Fax 49 (0) 7044-9445-722
www.camlog.de

L.D. Caulk Company, Dentsply, International
38 West Clarke Avenue
Milford, DE 19963-0359, USA
Phone (800) 532-2855
Fax (800) 788-4110
www.caulk.com

Central Florida Tissue Bank
8663 Commodity Circle
Orlando, FL 32819, USA
Phone (800) 852-0346; (407) 226-3888
Fax (407) 226-3885
www.tissuebank.org

CollaGenex Pharmaceuticals, Inc.
41 University Drive
Newtown, PA 18940, USA
Phone (215) 579-7388
Fax (215) 579-8577
www.collagenex.com

Columbia Scientific/Materialise Dental, Inc.
810-X Cromwell Park Drive
Glen Burnie, MD 21061, USA
Phone (888) 327-8202; (443) 557-0121
Fax (443) 557-0036
www.materialise.com

Columbus Dental
1000 Chouteau Avenue
St. Louis, MO 63188, USA
Phone (800) 325-7357

C.V. Mosby/Elsevier, Inc.
11830 Westline Industrial Drive
St. Louis, MO 63146, USA
Phone (800) 545-2522; (314) 872-8370
Fax (800) 535-9935; (314) 432-1280
www.elsevier.com

DENTSPLY Friadent CeraMed
12860 West Cedar Drive, Suite 110
Lakewood, CO 80228, USA
Phone (800) 426-7836; (303) 985-0800
Fax (303) 989-5669
www.dentsplyfc.com

DENTSPLY Friadent GmbH
Steinzeugstrasse 50
68229 Mannheim, GERMANY
Phone (49) 621-4302-000
Fax (40) 0621-4302-001
www.friadent.de

DENTSPLY Prosthetics Division
570 West College Avenue
York, PA 17405-0872, USA
Phone (808) 877-0020
Fax (717) 854-2343
http://prosthetics.dentsply.com

Designs for Vision, Inc.
760 Koehler Avenue
Ronkonkoma, NY 11779, USA
Phone (800) 727-6407; (631) 585-3300
Fax (631) 585-3404
www.designsforvision.com

DiskImplant
Victory S.A.
Rue la Martine 11
06000 Nice, FRANCE

Friadent USA; Inc.
Also See DENTSPLY Friadent CeraMed

Geistlich Pharma AG
Division Biomaterials
Bahnhofstrasse 40
CH-6110 Wolhusen, SWITZERLAND
Phone 41 (41) 492 56 30
Fax 41 (41) 492 56 39
www.geistlich.com

GlaxoSmithKline
One Franklin Plaza
Philadelphia, PA 19101, USA
Phone (888) 825-5249; (215) 751-4638
Fax (919) 315-3344
www.gsk.com

Global Surgical Corporation
3610 Tree Court Industrial Boulevard
St. Louis, MO 61322-6622, USA
Phone (805) 861-3585; (636) 861-3388
Fax (636) 861-2969
www.globalsurgical.com

Henry Schein, Inc.
135 Duryea Road
Melville, NY 11747, USA
Phone (631) 843-5500; (631) 843-5325
Fax (631) 843-5676
www.henryschein.com

Impla-Med Implant Group of APM-Sterngold
13794 N.W. Fourth Street, Suite 209
Sunrise, FL 33325, USA
Phone (800) 421-7321; (305) 846-0226
Fax (305) 948-6081
www.sterngold.com

Impladent Ltd.
198-45 Foothill Avenue
Holliswood, NY 11423, USA
Phone (800) 526-9343
Fax (718) 464 9620
www.impladentltd.com

Implant Direct, LLC.
27030 Malibu Hills Road
Calabasas Hills, CA 91301, USA
Phone (818) 444-3333
Fax (818) 444-3400
www.implantdirect.com

Implant Innovations, Inc. – A BIOMET Company
4555 Riverside Drive
Palm Beach Gardens, FL 33410, USA
Phone (800) 342-5454; (561) 776-6700
Fax (561) 776-1272
www.biomet3i.com

Implant Tracking Systems, LLC.
47 Norwood Road
West Hartford, CT 06117, USA
Fax (425) 790-2942
http://implanttracker.com

IMTEC Corporation
2401 North Commerce
Ardmore, OK 73401-6324, USA
Phone (800) 879-9799; (580) 223-4456
Fax (800) 986-9574; (580) 223-4561
www.imtec.com

IMZ Dental Implant System
Also See Attachments International

Innova Corp.- Kerr Sybron Dental Specialties
522 University Avenue, Suite 1200
Toronto, Ontario M5G 1W7, CANADA
Phone (800) 898-6261; (416) 340-8818
Fax (416) 340-0415
www.innovalife.com

Interpore Cross International –
A BIOMET Company
181 Technology Drive
Irvine, CA 92618, USA
Phone (949) 453-3200
Fax (949) 453-3225
www.interpore.com

KaVo Dental Corporation
340 East Route 22
Lake Zurich, IL 60047, USA
Phone (800) 323-8029; (847) 550-6800
Fax (847) 550-6825
www.kavousa.com

Kerr/Sybron Dental Specialties
1717 West Collins
Orange, CA 92867, USA
Phone (800) 537-7123; (714) 516-7400
Fax (800) 537-7345; (714) 516-7635
http://kerrdental.com

KLS Martin, L.P.
11239-1 St.Johns Industrial Parkway S.
Jacksonville, FL 32246-7652, USA
Phone (904) 641-7746; (800) 625-1557
Fax (904) 641-7378
www.klsmartinusa.com

Lifecore Biomedical, Inc.
(Formerly Implant Support Systems, Inc.)
Oral Restorative Division
3515 Lyman Boulevard
Chaska, MN 55318-3051, USA
Phone (800) 752-2663; (952) 368-4300
Fax (800) 651-8521; (952) 368-3411
www.lifecore.com

Luitpold Pharmaceuticals, Inc.
Osteohealth Company
One Luitpold Drive
Shirley, NY 11967, USA
Phone (800) 874-2334; (631) 924-4000
Fax (631) 924-1731
www.luitpold.com

Maxillon Laboratories, Inc.
P.O. Box 850, Hollis, NH 03049-0850, USA
Phone (888) 629-4566, (603) 594-9300
Fax (603) 594-9399
www.maxilon.com

Medesco Attachment Company
23461 South Point Drive
Laguna Hills, CA 92652-1523, USA
Phone (800) 633-3726
Fax (714) 588-9844

Medical Modelling, LLC
Also See AccuDental Guided Implant Modeling

Medizintechnik Gulden
Eschenweg 3
64397 Modautal, GERMANY
Phone 49 (0) 6254-94 38 40
Fax 49 (0) 6254-94 38 41
www.med-gulden.com

MMM – 3M ESPE Dental Products
3M Center Building 275-2SE-03
St. Paul, MN 55144-1000, USA
Phone (800) 634-2249
Fax (800) 728-0956
www.3mespe.com

Nobel Biocare USA, Inc.
22715 Savi Ranch Parkway
Yorba Linda, CA 92887, USA
Phone (800) 993-8100; (714) 282-4800
Fax (714) 998-9236
www.nobelbiocare.com

OCO Biomedical, Inc.
8500 Washington St., NE, Suite A-1
Albuquerque, NM 87113, USA
Phone (800) 228-0477; (505) 293-0025
Fax (505) 293-0447
www.ocobiomedical.com

Oral-B Laboratories, Inc.
Prudential Tower Building
Boston, MA 02199-8004, USA
Phone (617) 421-7000
www.oralb.com

Orascoptic, Inc.
3225 Deming Way, Suite 190
Middleton, WI 53562, USA
Phone (800) 369-3698; (608) 831-2555
Fax (608) 828-5265
www.orascoptic.com

Osseous Technologies of America
4500 Campus Drive, Suite 662
Newport Beach, CA 92660, USA
Phone (866) 901-5050
Fax (949) 250-0184
www.osseoustech.com

OsteoHealth, Co.
One Luitpold Drive
Shirley, NY 11967, USA
Phone (800) 874-2334; (631) 924-4000
Fax (631) 924-1731
www.osteohealth.com

Osteo-Implant Corporation
2415 Wilmington Road
New Castle, PA 16105-1956, USA
Phone (800) 654-5560; (724) 658-5321
Fax (724) 654-7640

Osteo-Med Corporation
3885 Arapaho Road
Addison, TX 75001, USA
Phone (800) 456-7779; (972) 677-4600
Fax (972) 677-4601
www.osteomedcorp.com

Pacific Coast Software, Inc.
23470 Olivewood Plaza Drive, Suite 240
Moreno Valley, CA 92553, USA
Phone (888) 263-3556
Fax (909) 243-6178

Pacific Coast Tissue Bank
2500-19 South Flower Street
Los Angeles, CA 90007, USA
Phone (213) 745-5560
Fax (213) 745-3031

Panadent Corporation
22573 Barton Road
Grand Terrace, CA 92313, USA
Phone (800) 368-9777; (909) 783-1841
Fax (909) 783-1896
www.panadent.com

Park Dental Research
19 West 34th Street, Suite 301
New York, NY 10001, USA
Phone (800) 243-7372; (212) 736-3765
Fax (212) 268-6845
www.parkdentalresearch.com

Periodontal Health Brush (PHB, Inc.)
P.O. Box 668
Osseo, WI 54758-9116, USA
Phone (800) 553-1440; (715) 597-3935
Fax (715) 597-3802
www.phbinc.com

Pfizer, Inc.
235 East 42nd Street
New York, NY 10017, USA
Phone (212) 733-2323
www.pfizer.com

Preat Corp.
2976 Long Valley Road
Santa Ynez, CA 93460, USA
Phone (800) 232-7732; (805) 693-8666
Fax (805) 693-8106
www.preat.com

Proctor & Gamble Distributing, Co.
1 Proctor & Gamble Plaza
C6-172, Box 36, Cincinnati, OH 45202, USA
Phone (513) 983-1100
Fax (513) 983-9369
www.pg.com

Pro-Dentec
(Professional Dental Technologies, Inc.)
PO Box 4160, Batesville, AR 72501, USA
Phone (870) 698-2300
Fax (870) 793-5554
www.prodentec.com

Quintessence Publishing Co., Inc.
4350 Chandler Drive
Hanover Park, IL 60133, USA
Phone (800) 621-0387; (630) 736-3600
Fax (630) 736-3633
www.quintpub.com

Raintree Essix, Inc.
4001 Division Street
Metairie, LA 70002, USA
Phone (800) 883-8733; (504) 488-0080
Fax (504) 488-2429
www.essix.com

Rapid Injection System Corp.
40 Roselle Street
Mineola, NY 11501, USA
Phone (516) 746-2622
Fax (516) 741-8147

Rhein'3 USA, Inc.
132 Monroe Street
Hoboken, NJ 07030, USA
Phone (877) 778-8383; (201) 217-0440
Fax (201) 217-0660
www.rhein83.com

Rocky Mountain Tissue Bank
2993 South Peoria Street, Suite 390
Aurora, CO 80014, USA
Phone (800) 424-5169; (303) 337-3330
Fax (303) 337-9383
www.rmtb.org

Salvin Dental Specialties, Inc.
3450 Latrobe Drive
Charlotte, NC 28211-4847, USA
Phone (800) 535-6566; (704) 442-5400
Fax (704) 442-5424
www.salvin.com

Sandoz, Inc.
506 Carnegie Center Drive, Suite 400
Princeton, NJ 08540, USA
Phone (800) 525-8747; (609) 627-8500
Fax (609) 627-8659
www.us.sandoz.com

Sargon Dental Implants
16101 Ventura Boulevard, Suite 350
Encino, CA 91436, USA
Phone (888) 688-6684; (818) 380-09050
Fax (818) 380-9059
www.sargondentalimplants.com

W. B. Saunders Company
The Curtis Center, Independence Square West
Philadelphia, PA 19106-3399, USA
Phone (215) 238-7800
Fax (215) 238-7883

Septodont, Inc.
245-C Quigley Boulevard
New Castle, DE 19720, USA
Phone (800) 872-8305
Fax (302) 328-5653
www.septodontinc.com

Sonicare
c/o Philips Domestic Appliances & Personal Care
1010 Washington Boulevard
Stamford, CT 06912, USA
Phone (800) 682-7664
www.sonicare.com

Sterngold/Sterngold Dental, LLC
23 Frank Mossberg Drive
Attleboro, MA 02703-0967, USA
Phone (800) 243-9942; (508) 226-5660
Fax (800) 531-2685; (508) 222-3593
www.sterngold.com

Straumann Holding AG
Peter Merian-Weg 12
CH-4002 Basel
SWITZERLAND
Phone 41 (61) 965 11 11
Fax 41 (61) 965 11 01
www.straumann.com

Tekscan, Inc.
307 West First Street
South Boston, MA 02127-1309, USA
Phone (800) 248-3669; (617) 464-4500
Fax (617) 464-4266
www.tekscan.com

Tel-Med Technologies
P.O. Box 595852
Fort Gratiot, MS 48059, USA
Phone (800) 243-4145
Fax (810) 987-4909

Teledyne Water Pik
1730 East Prospect Road
Fort Collins, CO 80553-0001, USA
Phone (800) 525-2774; (800) 854-9316

Thommen Medical USA, LLC.
Idea Center
1375, Euclid Avenue
Cleveland, OH 44115, USA
Phone (866) 319-9800
Fax (216) 583-9801
www.thommenmedical.com

Universal Implant Systems, Inc.
4400 Jennifer Street, N.W., Suite 220
Washington, DC 20015, USA
Phone (202) 244-9200
Fax (202) 244-3277

Walter Lorenz Surgical Instruments, Inc.
1520 Tradeport Drive
Jacksonville, FL 32218-2480, USA
Phone (904) 741-4400; (800) 874-7711
Fax (904) 741-4500; (904) 741-5521
www.lorenzsurgical.com

Warner Chilcott
100 Enterprise Drive
Rockaway, NJ 07866, USA
Phone (973) 442-3200
Fax (973) 442-3283
www.warnerchilcott.com

Zest Anchors, Inc.
2061 Wineridge Place, Suite 100
Escondido, CA 92029, USA
Phone (800) 262-2310; (760) 743-7744
Fax (800) 487-1357; (760) 743-7975
www.zestanchors.com

Zimmer Dental
1900 Aston Avenue
Carlsbad, CA 92008-7308, USA
Phone (800) 854-7019; (760) 929-4300
Fax (760) 431-7811
www.zimmerdental.com